W0254334

Cholesterol Systems in Insects and Animals

Editor

Jacqueline Dupont, Ph.D.
Department of Food and Nutrition
Iowa State University
Ames, Iowa

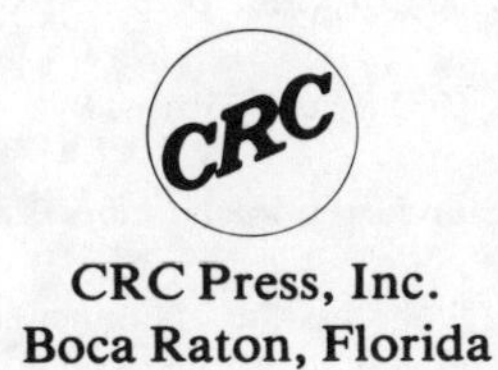

CRC Press, Inc.
Boca Raton, Florida

Library of Congress Cataloging in Publication Data

Main entry under title:

Cholesterol systems in insects and animals.

Bibliography
Includes index.
1. Insects—Physiology. 2. Cholesterol—
Metabolism. I. Dupont, Jacqueline, 1934-
QL495.C48 591.1'33 82-1355
ISBN 0-8493-5315-7 AACR

Direct all inquiries to CRC Press, Inc., 2000 Corporate Blvd., N.W., Boca Raton, Florida, 33431.

International Standard Book Number 0-8493-5315-7

Library of Congress Card Number 82-1355
Printed in the United States

PREFACE

There have been many conferences, monographs, books, and reviews about the myriad aspects of sterols and steroids during the past twenty-five years. Developments in knowledge of particular aspects of cholesterol metabolism have been very rapid and these have been reviewed regularly.

The reviews in this collection are unique in their intent to provide a basis for understanding of the subject. They include historical, descriptive, and comparative information which is not always presented in "state of the science" reviews. Cholesterol is viewed in each chapter as a part of a system — structural, kinetic, or metabolic. The complex nature of the place of cholesterol in living systems is illustrated in each chapter.

Each author has freely interpreted present information, selecting material which contributes to the understanding of current knowledge. The result is intended to provide an introduction to the subjects discussed which those not engaged in intensive research on one of the aspects may find useful.

The Editor is grateful to the authors who contributed to this volume. They have been patient and perseverant. The reviews represent years of study and thought by each contributor. Thanks are due to the illustrator, Donna Erickson, and to assistance from numerous others who helped each of us.

This work is the outcome of collaboration with colleagues and students over a professional lifetime. Credit is due to all who have contributed their work, thought, arguments, and kindnesses both in long association and occasional conversion. My enduring appreciation and respect is extended to all of those people.

EDITOR

Jacqueline Dupont, Ph.D., is the Chairman of the Department of Food and Nutrition, Iowa State University, Ames, Iowa.

Dr. Dupont received her B.S. degree in Food and Nutrition from Florida State University, her M.S. degree in Nutrition from Iowa State University, and obtained her Ph.D. in Food and Nutrition from Florida State University.

In addition to her current position, Dr. Dupont has held teaching and research positions with the USDA at Beltsville, Maryland, the Biochemistry Department of Howard University College of Medicine, and the Department of Food Science and Nutrition at Colorado State University.

Dr. Dupont is an active member of several professional organizations. These include the honorary organizations Omicron Nu, Sigma Xi, Phi Kappa Phi, and the New York Academy of Sciences. She is also a member of American Oil Chemists' Society American Dietetic Association, and the American Society of Clinical Nutrition. She is a Fellow of the American Heart Association Council on Arteriosclerosis.

She is the author of approximately 50 journal articles, as well as several chapters in books. Dr. Dupont's present research regards cholesterol and bile acid metabolism in the whole animal and dietary factors affecting regulation. She is also investigating essential fatty acids and prostaglandins.

CONTRIBUTORS

Satindra K. Goswami, Ph.D.
Department of Food Science
Cornell University
Ithaca, New York

Henry W. Kircher, Ph.D.
Professor
Department of Nutrition and Food Science
University of Arizona
Tuscon, Arizona

S. Y. Oh, Ph.D.
Director
Nutrition Research Institute
Oregon State University
Corvallis, Oregon

Rosemarie Ostwald, Ph.D.
Professor
Department of Nutrition
University of California at Berkeley
Berkeley, California

TABLE OF CONTENTS

Chapter 1

STEROLS AND INSECTS

Henry W. Kircher

TABLE OF CONTENTS

I. INTRODUCTION

Most animals are insects. Because of their small size, they are usually not as apparent as other organisms, but in numbers, insects are estimated to comprise 70 to 80% of all animal species and perhaps exist in more species than all other animal and plant species combined. Their habitats are extremely diverse, ranging from aquatic species in pools at the edge of glaciers to carnivores buried in the flesh of mammals.

Insects arose from some terrestrial arthropod about 250 to 300 million years ago. Their general form and life processes have remained largely unaltered for the last 150 million years. Fossil records of cockroaches show that little morphological change occurred in some species over this period. Many climatological and geological changes took place during this time; the present ubiquity of cockroaches is a good reflection of their past adaptive potential.

Insects are one of the few multicellular organisms that still use *Homo sapiens* as prey. Insects can see, hear, feel, smell, taste, eat, digest, excrete, reproduce bisexually, fly, and walk upside down. Some are viviparous and parthenogenic. They go through several discrete life stages — egg, embryo, larva, and pupa — during which the nymph, maggot, grub, or caterpillar tissues differentiate into wings, legs, gonads, eyes, antennae, and sex organs. Finally, the reproductive adult form emerges to start a new life cycle.

The principal aspect of the life of insects that is of interest here, however, is their inability to synthesize cholesterol. The tissues of all other animals higher than nematodes in the evolutionary scale and of all plants beyond certain bacteria can assemble isoprene units to squalene and cyclize the latter to lanosterol or cycloartenol. These two tetracyclic triterpenes are then further metabolized by living systems to hundreds of naturally occurring sterol molecules: phytosterols, sapogenins, cardenolides, steroid alkaloids, sex hormones, corticoids, and bile acids. Insects, although able to metabolize ingested sterols, cannot synthesize them *de novo*.

The discovery that insects require a dietary sterol for growth and maturation took place in the middle 1930s. Hobson[1] and Van't Hoog,[2] working with a blow fly and a fruit fly, found that the addition of cholesterol to organic solvent extracted media ingredients restored the nutritional value of the diets and allowed the insects to go through their full life cycle. In the absence of the sterol, the flies died during the early larval stages.

During the next two decades, numerous other insects were tested with essentially the same results.[3] A sterol free diet inhibited growth and usually caused larval death. All common sterols with an intact skeleton and a 3β-hydroxy group were utilized to varying degrees. Some sterol esters were used, others were not. Hydroxylation of the B ring at C-6 or C-7 or truncation of the side chain to cholane, pregnane, or androstane derivatives prevented their use. By 1956, the following observations were generally accepted:

1. Insects required an exogenous source of sterol. It is principally supplied by the diet, but may also come from intestinal microorganisms.
2. Cholesterol can be universally used.
3. Plant eating insects can also use phytosterols, e.g., ergosterol, sitosterol, stigmasterol; carnivorous species, such as the hide beetle, appeared to require cholesterol.
4. The ability to use various sterols and the dietary concentrations required for optimal growth varies between species.

Results reported by the early workers on sterol utilization should be viewed with care. The criteria used in most of the studies were limited to rates of larval development, the size of the insect, and its ability to pupate. Reproductive capacity was rarely measured. The purity of phytosterols was also difficult to assess, and often the sources of the sterols and their physical constants were not reported. Commercially available sitosterol, for instance, contained as much as 40% campesterol as an impurity. In addition, it was not realized that female insects transferred essential sterols to their progeny through the egg, thus allowing the young to mature on diets containing inadequate sterols.

During the next eight years, a number of discoveries and new observations became the basis for much of the recent progress in research dealing with insects and sterols.[4] With the use of labeled compounds, gas and thin-layer chromatography, it was shown in several insects that neither acetate, mevalonate, nor squalene was metabolized to sterols. From these studies, the dogma that insects lack the enzyme systems for sterol biosynthesis became well established and has never been refuted. The "sparing sterol" concept, speculations on the functions of sterols in insects, and the first concrete demonstration of the metabolism of an ingested sterol by an insect were published at this time.[5-7] The insect molting hormone, ecdysone, was shown to be derived from dietary cholesterol and to be a pentahydroxy-Δ^7-6-keto derivative of this sterol.[8,9]

Since 1965, all of these facets, as well as several new developments, continue to stimulate investigations of the relationships between sterols and insects. These relationships are discussed in the remainder of this chapter.

II. ABSENCE OF STEROL SYNTHESIS BY INSECTS

Early nutritional studies provided indirect evidence that insects lack the enzyme systems needed for sterol biosynthesis. Subsequent work with labeled precursors showed this to be true. Larvae of the hide beetle were reared on diets that contained ^{14}C-acetate or ^{14}C-fructose and the lipids isolated from the insects.[5] No ^{14}C was found in either case in the carefully purified squalene and sterols obtained from the beetles. In addition, mevalonic acid, squalene, lanosterol, and 4,4′-dimethyl-8-cholestenol were all unable to replace dietary cholesterol. From this, Clark and Bloch[5] concluded that the sterol biosynthetic pathway was multiply blocked in insects. Similar studies with other species gave the same result.[4] The isolation of radioactive sterol from the silverfish after it had eaten ^{14}C-acetate with its diet[10] is now considered to be the result of sterol synthesis by intestinal microorganisms. Even intracellular microorganisms, capable of supplying their host with sterols, have recently been discovered in tissues of the smaller brown plant hopper.[11] Administration of ^{14}C-acetate to a primitive insect, the firebrat, either by diet or injection failed to yield any radioactive sterols.[12]

Later studies with spiders, millipedes, prawns, crabs, and lobsters showed that these animals were also unable to convert ^{14}C-acetate to sterols.[13,14] It is now generally accepted that the capability of sterol biosynthesis is lacking throughout the phylum Arthropoda. Since insects are believed to have evolved from an earlier arthropod, they have probably been unable to synthesize sterols during their entire existence on earth.

III. UTILIZATION OF STEROLS BY INSECTS

The nutritional value of various sterols to insects was already considered by the first investigators. Both Hobson[1] and Van't Hoog[2] recognized that the insects' response was affected by the structure of the dietary sterol. In both cases, cholesterol appeared to be satisfactory. The two plant sterols, sitosterol and ergosterol, were equivalent to cholesterol for the fruit fly[2] but less effective than cholesterol for promoting the growth of a blow fly.[1] Similar nutritional experiments performed on other species[3,4] led to the concepts of sterol "utilization" by insects and sterol "requirements" of insects.

These are commonly assessed by a correlation of the structure and concentration of one or two sterols in the diet with some parameter in the life cycle of the insect. Larval growth, pupation, adult emergence (eclosion), and reproduction have all been used as criteria. A sterol deficient diet is devised that is adequate in all other nutrients and various sterols are added to it. The efficacy of the test sterols for growth promotion, pupation, or reproduction is determined by comparisons to the insects' performance on control diets. These usually contain no added sterol or cholesterol. The comparisons are then used to classify the test sterols as (1) usable, they fulfill the sterol requirements of the insect; (2) less effective than a control (usually cholesterol); or (3) not usable, the performance of the insect is the same as on the test diet with no added sterol.

The tolerance of insects to dietary sterol concentrations varies tremendously. Oriental house fly larvae are not affected by as much as 15% cholesterol in their diet, whereas 6.3% was fatal to a seed weevil;[15] 0.013% dietary cholesterol was optimal for the common house fly[16] and only 4 mg of the sterol in 100 mℓ of medium was deleterious to the first two stages of the cabbage root fly.[17] The adult forms of most insects tested had no dietary sterol requirements except for reproduction. A cockroach could be kept alive for almost two years on a sterol free diet,[4] but the adult boll weevil needed at least 20 mg of cholesterol per 100 g diet for normal longevity (55 to 89 days). On sterol-free diets, the weevils died in about two weeks.[18]

Most of the work that has been done to date (July 81) on insect sterol nutrition is summarized in Table 1. Various aspects of the data are discussed after the table.

Table 1
THE UTILIZATION OF STEROLS AND RELATED COMPOUNDS BY INSECTS

Number of insect species tested (Refs. in parenthesis)

Compound	Compound was: Used	Less Effective	Not used
Common sterols			
Cholesterol	47 (1,2,4,5,15-43c)	1 (44,45)	5 (17,46-49)
Sitosterol	3 (4,17,19,21,22,24, 29-33,35,37-39,41, 43c,44-46,50-53)	4 (1,2,15,20,43a)	5 (6,19,25,28,42,43, 48,54)
7-Dehydrocholesterol	18 (19,22,30,32,33,37,39, 43)	3 (15,31,43a)	7 (4,20,21,35,38,43c)
Ergosterol	18 (2,4,7,19,22,30,32,37, 39,47,49)	7 (1,4,15,20, 31,45)	11 (6,19,21,22,25,33,35, 38,41-44,48)
Cholestanol	12 (4,19,21,22,30,32, 38,39)	8 (2,19,31,37, 43a,c)	11 (4,6,15,18,19,22,23, 36,40,45,55,56)
Stigmasterol	12 (4,20,22,30,32,33,37, 38,41,43c,51)	5 (2,4,15,31,44, 45)	4 (6,21,42,43,48)
Cholesteryl acetate	10 (15,19-21,30,32,53)	1 (45)	—
Other cholesteryl esters	4 5315 (15,20,30,53)	—	4 (20,43a,45,53)
Campesterol	6 (28,35,41,51,52,57,58)	2 (42,43c)	—
Desmosterol	7 (5,24,29,53,59,60)	1 (37)	3 (37,59,61)
Zymosterol	2 (19,22)	1 (19)	8 (4,19,22)
Less common sterols			
C27			
Cholest-4-en-3β-ol	1 (15)	—	2 (4,37)
22-Dehydrocholesterol	1 (53)	—	1 (6)
Lathosterol	1 (48)	2 (37,43c)	2 (6,37)
Coprostanol	1 (4)	—	1 (37)
7-Coprostenol	—	—	1 (37)
3α or 3β-Chlorocholesterols	—	—	4 (2,15,30,37)
3-Keto-cholesterols	1 (2)	1 (15)	7 (16,20,21,22,37,38,40)
Cholestane, cholest-5-ene	—	—	9 (15,19,20,22,30,32)
3α-Hydroxycholesterols	1 (4)	—	2 (2,15,37)
7-Hydroxy, 7-Ketocholesterols	—	—	10 (15,19,21,22)
24-Hydroxy, 24-Ketocholesterols	—	—	1 (24,41)
6-Ketocholestanol, cholesteryl methyl ether, cholestan-3β,5α,6β-triol	—	—	2 (30,37)
Cholesta-5,23,24-trien-3β-ol	—	—	1 (62)
C28			
Ergostanol	—	1 (20)	—
7-Ergostenol	—	—	2 (6,48)
7,22-Ergostadienol	—	—	1 (6)
5,7-Ergostadienol	—	—	1 (6)
Brassicasterol	1 (52)	1 (43c)	1 (43)
Dihydrobrassicasterol	1 (52)	—	1 (57)
24-Methylenechol	3 (24,41,52,60)	1 (37)	—
24-Methylenecholesterol 24,28-epoxide	—	—	1 (41)
C29			
Stigmastanol	1 (4)	—	—
Schottenol	1 (48)	1 (43c)	—
Clionasterol	1 (131b)	1 (16)	1 (43)
Spinasterol	—	1 (43c)	—

Table 1 (continued)
THE UTILIZATION OF STEROLS AND RELATED COMPOUNDS BY INSECTS

Number of insect species tested (Refs. in parenthesis)

Compound	Compound was: Used	Less Effective	Not used
Fucosterol	3 (24,41,52,53)	—	—
Isofucosterol	1 (24,41)	—	—
Fucosterol 24,28-epoxide	1 (24,41)	—	—
28-Keto, 28-Keto-24-hydroxy,24,28-Dihydroxysitosterols	—	—	1 (24,41)
Stigmasta-5,24(28),28-trien-3β-ol	—	—	1 (62)
24,28-Iminofucosterol	—	—	1 (63)
Sterol precursors, nor-sterols, metabolites			
Mevalonic acid	—	—	3 (5,30,45)
Squalene	—	—	6 (5,21,30,32,35,45)
Lanosterol	—	—	6 (5,21,30,32,35,47)
4,4′-Dimethyl-8-cholestenol	—	—	1 (5)
Lophenol	—	—	2 (48,56)
Calciferol, Ergocalciferol	—	—	12 (2,15,19,21,30,37,45,47)
Lumisterol	—	—	2 (2,47)
Bile acids, Androgens, Estrogens, Progestagens	—	—	7 (2,15,21,30,37,38,43c)
25-Norcholesterol	—	1 (37)	—
Nor-and Bisnorcholesteryl acetates	—	1 (64)	—

A. Common Sterols

1. Cholesterol

For thirty years after the discovery of the dietary requirement of sterols by insects, it was found that cholesterol could fulfill this function for every insect that was tested. In fact it appeared to be the optimal sterol for all except the silkworm, which could use cholesterol but grew better on a diet that contained sitosterol, the principal sterol in mulberry leaves.[44] In 1965, a fruit fly, *Drosophila pachea,* was discovered that could not use cholesterol or any of the common sterols.[48] The adaptation of *D. pachea* to the alkaloid and Δ^7-sterol rich senita cactus in the Sonoran desert of Arizona and northwestern Mexico probably resulted in the loss of this species' ability to use sterols with only a Δ^5 double bond.[65-67]

Since then, cholesterol was shown to be ineffective or deleterious as the sole dietary sterol in certain life stages of four other insects. The moth *Crambus trisectus* was unable to use cholesterol; it required sitosterol in its diet.[46] The fungus feeding ambrosia beetle could use dietary cholesterol for larval maturation or egg laying by the female but needed a $\Delta^{5,7}$-sterol such as ergosterol or 7-dehydrocholesterol for pupation.[47] Cholesterol in the diet also decreased locomotor activity, reproduction, and life span of this insect compared to the two $\Delta^{5,7}$ sterols.[47a] Cholesterol was not a suitable dietary sterol for the tea tortrix; it also required dietary ergosterol to complete its life cycle.[49] Young larvae of the cabbage root fly are very sensitive to modest concentrations of cholesterol.[17] Addition of as little as 3 mg of cholesterol to 100 mℓ of its diet, only about one tenth of the normal sterol concentration in insect diets, significantly increased larval mortality and halved the weight of the survivors when compared to controls. During the later larval stages of this insect, however, media with as much as 400 mg of cholesterol in 100 mℓ of the diet had no harmful effect on the larvae or their subsequent development into adults.[17] However, cholesterol is an adequate dietary sterol for most insects and is normally used by entomologists in the development of chemically defined diets.

2. Cholestanol, the "Sparing Sterol" Concept, and Ovarian Transfer of Sterols to Progeny

The utilization of cholestanol by insects is still an open question.[55] Cholestanol is not a constituent of the food eaten by insects and there are no problems of interpretation in those cases where this sterol cannot be used (11 species, Table 1). The results obtained in the remaining examples, however, need to be considered together with two series of observations. One of these led to the "sparing sterol" concept, and the other to the discovery that some insects transfer significant quantities of sterols to their progeny via eggs.

The sparing sterol concept was developed by Clark and Block[6] in their work with the hide beetle. This carnivorous insect required at least 1 mg of cholesterol in 6 g diet for pupation; the larvae failed to mature and died with only 0.25 or 0.5 mg of cholesterol per 6 g diet. Cholestanol, lathosterol, 22-dehydro-cholesterol, sitosterol, or 7-ergostenol all failed to provide for larval development. When 1 mg of these sterols and 0.25 mg of cholesterol were added to 6 g diet, the larvae grew and pupated as readily as on the 1 mg cholesterol diet. In one experiment, only 0.03 mg of cholesterol plus 1 mg of sitosterol was nutritionally equivalent to 1 mg of cholesterol. From this, Clark and Block concluded that the other sterols satisfy a relatively nonspecific requirement for sterol in the insect and "spare" the small amount of cholesterol in the diet for metabolic or hormonal purposes. A "sparing sterol" is therefore one which is inadequate when it is the only sterol in the diet, but provides for normal growth and development when subminimal quantities of an essential sterol are also present.

In a later paper, many sterols were tested for their sparing capacity in the hide beetle.[60] The sparing sterols all had a 3β-hydroxy group, a Δ^5-double bond or a 5α-A/B ring junction, but not all sterols which had these structural features were sparing. Stigmastanol and fucosterol were only slightly active; ergosterol and 22-stigmastenol were without any sparing activity. Cholestanol was subsequently shown to be a sparing sterol also for the boll weevil,[18] house fly,[40] blow fly,[36] fruit fly,[55] and two cockroaches[23,68] when used in diets containing inadequate quantities of cholesterol.

The transfer of sterols from females to their progeny was first demonstrated with house flies. Cholesterol was required for egg production,[69] and ^{14}C-cholesterol injected into adult females or eaten during the larval stages was not excreted, but later placed into their eggs.[70,71] Similar results were observed with the ambrosia beetle. If the female is on a diet that contains ergosterol, enough of this sterol is transferred in the eggs to the progeny so that these larvae can pupate even though they are on a $\Delta^{5,7}$-sterol free diet.[72]

Recent studies with axenic *D. melanogaster* clarified the cholestanol-cholesterol interplay in this insect.[55] Flies could be reared from a cholestanol medium if their maternal parent had cholesterol in its food. Sufficient cholesterol was transmitted through the egg so that cholestanol acted as a sparing sterol. When these cholestanol reared F_1 adults were then allowed to oviposit on cholesterol, cholestanol or sterol free media, 84%, 0.5%, and 0.6% of their eggs, respectively, gave rise to F_2 adults.

In another experiment, the F_1 adults from the cholestanol medium were placed on cholesterol medium for several days. They were intermittently removed from this to oviposit on fresh cholestanol medium. Within 2 days after feeding on the cholesterol medium, the females incorporated enough of this sterol into their eggs so that their progeny could go to F_2 adults on the cholestanol medium.[55]

The data for cholestanol in Table 1 should now be considered in the light of these findings. It is possible that the 19 species that were able to utilize this sterol were using it as a "sparing sterol" and were able to get sufficient quantities of a requisite Δ^5-sterol as an impurity in the "sterol-free" diet or via the egg. Before a sterol such as cholestanol is classified to be nutritionally adequate as the sole dietary sterol for an insect, at least two and preferably three generations should be reared from media that contain it.

3. 7-Dehydrocholesterol

This sterol has been detected as a metabolite of cholesterol in several insects (*vide infra*) and can be used by most species that were tested (Table 1). In some cases, the free sterol, but not its benzoate, could be used.[19] It was less effective than cholesterol in the diet of a house fly[15] and flesh fly,[31] and could not be used at all by the mosquito,[4] pine beetle,[35] German cockroach,[20] two locusts,[21] and the corn earworm.[43c] These last five insects were also unable to use ergosterol, the principal $\Delta^{5,7}$-sterol in nature.

4. Ergosterol

This common sterol in the diet of yeast and fungus feeding insects can also be used by many species that do not normally feed on microorganisms. It has been classified as less effective than cholesterol for several phytophagous and omnivorous insects (Table 1), and in this capacity, may be acting as a sparing sterol. In addition to the five insects mentioned under 7-dehydrocholesterol, ergosterol could not be used by three carnivorous insects,[19,22,25] the silkworm,[44] corn borer,[33] *D. pachea*,[48] and the corn earworm.[43c] The available evidence suggests that in these four cases, the presence of the 24β-methyl group rather than the $\Delta^{5,7}$-diene system in ergosterol prevents its utilization. However, no 5,7,22-trienes other than ergosterol have been tested as yet.

5. Sitosterol, Stigmasterol, and Campesterol

These are the three principal sterols in the food of most phytophagous insects and can be used by almost all that have been tested. A few exceptions exist, however. Adults of the cotton leafworm failed to lay viable eggs when 0.1% sitosterol was incorporated into their diet of yeast and dry kidney beans.[54] This is hard to rationalize because sitosterol is the principal sterol in cotton.[73-75] Stigmasterol was not used by two species of locust[21] and was reported to be less effective than sitosterol for the silkworm.[44] Campesterol could be used by all seven species tested (Table 1). Neither sitosterol nor stigmasterol were used by two carnivorous insects,[6,25] or the omnivorous house fly.[28] The three sterols fed to worker bees provided fewer (48-65%) sealed brood progeny than cholesterol (100%).[28a] However no matter which sterol was added to the worker's diet, 24-methylenecholesterol was the principal sterol in the larvae. Worker bees probably furnished this sterol to the brood from sterols accumulated in their tissues before they were placed on the defined diets.[28b]

6. Cholesteryl Esters

Numerous insects can use cholesteryl acetate as readily as cholesterol as the sole dietary sterol (Table 1). In an extensive study with the omnivorous German cockroach, Noland[20] found that cholesteryl formate, acetate, butyrate, palmitate, benzoate, and dimethylacetate, as well as sitosteryl and stigmasteryl acetates, could all be used by the insect. Only cholesteryl trimethylacetate (pivalate) could not; it was presumably sterically too hindered to be hydrolyzed by the esterases of the cockroach.

In other cases, two beetles could use 7-dehydrocholesterol but not its benzoate;[19] the silkworm could use cholesteryl acetate but not the benzoate or stearate;[45] and the khapra beetle could use some, but not all of the many cholesteryl esters tested.[53] Two hymenopterous parasites were maintained with cholesteryl linoleate, but little growth occurred and mortality was high.[43a] No work has yet been reported with steryl glycosides or acylated steryl glycosides as the sole sterol ingredient in insect diets.

7. Desmosterol

This sterol is an intermediate in the dealkylation of phytosterols to cholesterol in several insects, and so it is reasonable to assume that all insects that are able to perform this dealkylation can use desmosterol. Phytophagous insects that have been reported to use desmosterol are the confused flour beetle,[59] tobacco hornworm,[29] fruit fly,[37] and silkworm,[24] as well as the omnivorous German and American cockroaches[59] and the carnivorous hide beetle[5] (however for conflicting results with the hide beetle see References 4 and 59). The use of this sterol may depend on the presence of a Δ^{24}-reductase in insects, an enzyme that is required in the biosynthesis of cholesterol by animals and plants.

8. Zymosterol

Most of the evidence obtained with this sterol suggests that it cannot be used by insects. In the two cases where it was reported to be used by beetles,[19,22] it may have acted as a sparing sterol. Unfortunately, other than the triterpene lanosterol, no other $\Delta^{8(9)}$-sterols have been tested. Until definitive studies are made, it can be assumed that insects lack the $\Delta^{8(9)}$-Δ^{7} isomerases present in other animals and plants.

B. Less Common Sterols

Nutritional experiments with these compounds were done with fewer insects than those in the preceding section, and in many cases, with only a single species. Some are important, however, for demonstrating how deviations from the structure of cholesterol render the compound unusable by insects. These include substitution of the 3β-hydroxyl group by chlorine, hydrogen, methoxyl, a 3α-hydroxyl group, a ketone, hydroxylation at carbons 5 and 6, oxidation at the 7-position, or a change of the double bond from Δ^{5} to Δ^{4}.

Little can be said about the other sterols in this section of Table 1; there is not enough evidence to draw broad conclusions. Lathosterol was required by *D. pachea;*[76] it could not be used by a strain of *D. melanogaster*[37] or the hide beetle.[6] The three $\Delta^{24(28)}$-sterols, 24-methylenecholesterol, fucosterol, and isofucosterol are intermediates in the dealkylation of phytosterols and were usable by the silkworm,[24] fruit fly,[37] and tobacco hornworm.[52] In some cases, nonutilization resulted from an inability of a carnivorous insect to dealkylate phytosterols.[6,31,43] Finally, the two side chain allenic derivatives, cholesta-5,23,24-trien-3β-ol and stigmasta-5,24(28),28-trien-3β-ol, were not only unusable by the silkworm, but the former inhibited growth and development even when a usable sterol such as sitosterol was also in the diet.[62]

C. Sterol Precursors, Nor-sterols and Metabolites

The sterol requirement of numerous insects could not be met by several of the intermediates in cholesterol biosynthesis (Table 1). Mevalonic acid, squalene, lanosterol, and 4,4′-dimethyl-8-cholestenol were not used nor did these compounds act as sparing sterols with a subminimal quantity of cholesterol in the diet.[5] The methyl group in lophenol prevented its use by two species of *Drosophila.*[48,56] Phytophagous insects can apparently remove a methyl group at C_{24} in the side chain but not from C_{4} in the A-ring of sterols.

The "less effective" utilization of various nor-cholesterols by the house fly[64] and *D. melanogaster*[37] is probably due to their sparing sterol activity in these insects. Steroids with severely truncated or modified side chains (bile acids, androgens, estrogens,

Table 2
FUNCTIONS OF STEROLS IN VERTEBRATES AND IN INSECTS

Function	Vertebrates	Insects
Membrane constituent	Cholesterol	Depends on dietary sterols
Hormones to control reproductive, metabolic, and maturation processes	Progestagens, androgens, estrogens, corticoids	Ecdysteroids
Defensive secretions	Bufadienolides (toad poisons)	Progestagens, androgens cardenolides, bufadienolides
Fat emulsifiers	Bile acids, bile alcohols	—
Calcium metabolism	Vitamin D	—

progestagens), or an opened B-ring (calciferol), cannot fulfill the sterol requirement of insects and do not act in a sparing sterol capacity.[6] The change in configuration of the C_{19}-methyl group from β (7-dehydrocholesterol) to α (lumisterol) also inhibited utilization of the latter by *D. melanogaster*[2] and the ambrosia beetle.[47]

D. Summary

Insects can use a wide variety of sterols in their diets. They appear to have an absolute requirement for a 3β-hydroxy group, a complete cholesterol side chain, and a Δ^5 double bond although exceptions to this exist. The ''essential sterol'' sparing ability of many other sterols and the transfer of sterols to progeny via the egg are two reasons why the results obtained in many of the experiments listed in Table 1 should be viewed with caution. A review on techniques for the isolation and identification of sterols in insects has recently appeared.[64a]

IV. STATUS AND FUNCTION OF STEROLS IN INSECTS

Sterols are used by insects, as they are by vertebrates, as essential components of biological membranes, in reproduction, as precursors for steroid hormones, and as defensive secretions. In contrast to vertebrates, however, insects do not appear to synthesize bile acids for lipid emulsification or hydroxylated cholecalciferols for calcium metabolism (Table 2). The utilization of dietary sterols for ecdysone biosynthesis and the various roles of the hormone in biochemical and biological processes is covered in a following section. Other functions of sterols in insects are discussed below.

A. Dietary Uptake and Tissue Distribution of Sterols

The structures and concentrations of sterols in insects are a function of the kinds of sterols in their diet, the ability of the insects to absorb and modify them, and the specific requirements of the various tissues and organs for these compounds.

1. Uptake

Selective uptake of dietary sterols was first reported for house flies.[77] Even though sitosterol was the principal sterol in the diet, campesterol, a minor component, constituted 74% of the flies' tissue sterols. When cholesterol was added to the diet, it became the principal tissue sterol (Table 3).

Similar results were observed with a cockroach.[78] Sterols were taken up predominately in the crop and sitosterol was absorbed half as efficiently as cholesterol from the diet. Cholesterol and cholestanol, however, possessing the same side chain, were absorbed equally well.[79] The Khapra beetle also selectively absorbs certain sterols from its diet; more than twice as much cholesterol and campesterol are found in its tissues

Table 3
DIETARY VS. PUPAL STEROLS OF THE HOUSE FLY[77]

	Pupal Sterols (%)		
	Campesterol	Sitosterol	Cholesterol
0.2% campesterol, 0.2% sitosterol	77	21	
0.2% campesterol, 0.2% cholesterol	19		77
0.2% sitosterol, 0.2% cholesterol		9	89
0.35% sitosterol, 0.15% campesterol	76	21	

as are in its food.[79a] In contrast, no selectivity was noted during the absorption of phytosterols by the milkweed bug; cholesterol, campesterol, sitosterol, and stigmasterol were recovered from the insect in almost the same proportions as they existed in the diet.[80]

Growth inhibition of the carnivorous hide beetle at 35% relative humidity (r.h.) by several plant sterols (sitosterol, stigmasterol, ergosterol) in the presence of adequate quantities of cholesterol was interpreted as an interference with cholesterol uptake by the larvae.[81] In a subsequent paper, the authors reported a reversal of this effect at 65% r.h., even though the phytosterols depressed the cholesterol content of the insects.[42] Apparently the beetle's requirement for cholesterol was higher at 35% r.h. than at 65% r.h.; the lower humidity is probably a more stressful condition.

Utilization of dietary sitosterol by the silkworm was greatly enhanced when fatty acids were added to the diet.[82] Perhaps the absorption of the sterol by the gut was facilitated by the acids either by ester or micelle formation. Little is known about possible synergistic effects which may occur between these two lipid constituents in the natural food of insects.

2. Tissue Sterols

Sterols are found in all tissues of insects, where they play principally a structural role. In one of the first studies, cholesterol occurred in 17 different tissues and organs of the American cockroach, ranging from 0.15 μg/mg in the cuticle to 1 μg/mg in the gut.[83] A cockroach reared on a diet containing 0.005% cholesterol and 0.1% cholestanol contained both sterols in all tissues.[23] Highest concentrations were again in the alimentary canal and also in the ventral nerve, where cholesterol was preferentially deposited. Almost all of the other tissues also contained a higher proportion of cholesterol in their sterol fraction than was present in the diet. Free sterols appear to predominate over esters in the hemolymph[84,85] and all cells[23,83] with some exceptions,[86,87] and are almost entirely associated with subcellular particulate fractions.[4] Sterol esters are probably storage forms; their concentrations are highest in fat body,[83] nerve tissues,[23,83] ovaries[88] and eggs.[71,89,90] The composition of tissue sterols reflects their composition in the diet together with selective uptake or excretion[77] as well as the ability of various insects to modify sterol structures by dealkylation, desaturation, or saturation of double bonds.[51] Based on experiments with sparing sterols, the requirements of tissues for sterols as structural components are not as specific as the needs of some tissues for sterols for metabolic purposes[6] or some very specific structural role.[23] The very slow turnover rates of carcass cholesterol with dietary ^{14}C-cholesterol[27] or cholestanol[79] suggest that some of the insects' sterols are tightly bound into discrete structures. It is apparent that cholesterol fills a niche of high structural specificity in certain tissues from which it cannot readily be displaced; this may be in the mitochondrial and endoplasmic reticular membranes.[79]

The relatively high ratio of cholesterol to cholestanol (1:1 to 2:1) in the nerve tissues of cockroaches reared on a diet containing a 1:19 ratio of the two sterols indicates a highly specific role for the unsaturated sterol in the myelin sheaths.[79,91] In another example, when house fly larvae were reared on a medium that was very deficient in cholesterol, the deficiency reduced growth and the sterol was taken up preferentially by the nervous system at the expense of other tissues.[92] House fly larvae also accumulate dietary cholesterol at a faster rate than they gain weight and convert very little of the sterol to esters, again showing the importance of free sterols to larval growth and development.[89]

Distribution of sterols in organs and tissues of a few other insects was reported. More cholesterol was found in the lipids of the muscles, reproductive organs, and guts of termites than in their fat bodies, and more in the lipids of the head than in the lipids of the thoraces or abdomens.[86] The cholesterol content of cricket hemolymph (blood) varied between 120 and 230 mg percent for female adults and larvae (both sexes), respectively. The sterol concentration remained about the same for males from the larval to adult stage, but dropped markedly in the adult female. This is probably due to the high degree of sterol incorporation into the egg.[85] The concentration of free sterols in maturing silkworm ovaries decreased a little (1 mg to 0.8 mg/g tissue), while the sterol ester concentration increased about fivefold (0.2 mg to 1 mg/g tissue).[88] This also correlates with the relatively high concentration of sterol ester in insect eggs.[90] Lipids were extracted from the hemolymph (1.16 mg/mℓ), guts, fat bodies, and integument of Mopani moth caterpillars. Sterols constituted 11% of the hemolymph lipids, 6.7% of gut lipids, and only 0.16% of fat body lipids. All were mixtures of cholesterol and dietary sterols.[93]

In contrast to typical phytophagous insects, which convert a portion of their dietary sterols to cholesterol, the composition of the carcass sterols of the milkweed bug is essentially the same as that in the diet,[80] and that of the Mexican bean beetle consists principally of stanols.[94,95] As yet, there are no rationales for these observations. Until synthetic diets are devised for these two insects and their various tissues are analyzed, it will be difficult to explain their unusual sterol compositions.

B. Sterols in Reproduction

1. Ovarian Development

Development of ovaries in female house flies held for six days on sugar water after adult emergence from the pupae depended on the presence of cholesterol in the larval diet. The ovarian tissue remained immature in the adult stage when cholesterol was omitted during the larval stage or was replaced by sitosterol.[96] Sitosterol is not dealkylated by house flies and cannot be used for reproduction by these insects.[28] Maturation of ovaries during silkworm development resulted in a steady increase of free sterols and a large proportional increase of sterol esters, rising from 0.2 to 1 mg of ester per gram ovarian tissue in 9 days.[88]

2. Oogenesis and Egg Laying

The importance of sterols for oogenesis was demonstrated with several insects. When ^{14}C-cholesterol was injected into adult house flies, very little label was excreted. Most of the compound was placed by the females into their eggs.[70] Addition of cholesterol to a house fly larval diet doubled subsequent egg production by the adults,[97] and larval dietary ^{14}C-cholesterol was deposited into eggs even after the adults were placed on a diet than contained nonradioactive sterol.[71] Both cholesteryl esters and 7-dehydrocholesterol were present in higher concentrations in house fly eggs than in the females which laid them.[71,90] The esters are probably storage forms of the sterols to be hydrolyzed during embryogenesis[89] and the 7-dehydrocholesterol may be present as a prohormone.[98] Females on a sterol-free medium placed up to 60% of their body sterols into their eggs, and the proportion of 7-dehydrocholesterol in the egg sterols rose from 16 to 37% even though the total sterol contents decreased as egg laying progressed and the females' tissue sterols were being depleted.[99]

Other insects required a constant dietary sterol intake for oogenesis. A cockroach could be kept alive on a sterol free diet, but egg production quickly ceased.[4] When adult *D. melanogaster* were placed on a minimal diet that contained 300 mg of cholesterol per liter, they laid 10 eggs per day per female; only 2 were laid in the absence of dietary sterol.[99a] In other work with the same species, one-week-old females reared through the larval stages on three media were maintained and allowed to oviposit for 24 hr on the same medium from which they were reared. Those on cholesterol laid on the average 52 eggs per individual, those on cholestanol, 31 eggs, and those on a sterol-free medium, 28 eggs. Dissection of the females showed fewer eggs in the ovaries of those reared on cholestanol than those from the cholesterol medium.[55]

Similar results had been observed with boll weevils, an insect that requires a daily intake of cholesterol for fertility. When adults that had been reared on a cholesterol medium were maintained on that medium, they laid 6 to 8 eggs per female per day. When placed on media containing the same concentration of cholestanol (40 mg/100 g diet) their egg production fell to zero as it did when they were placed on a medium that lacked a sterol.[18]

3. Embryogenesis and Hatchability

Although the absence of cholesterol in the diet of adult house flies had no effect on egg laying, the hatchability of the eggs soon decreased to nearly zero. Subsequent addition of cholesterol to the diet brought hatchability back to control levels within a short time.[69] The importance of a sterol during embryogenesis was demonstrated when 50% of the larvae hatching from eggs laid by adults reared from a cholesterol deficient medium did not mature even when the larvae were placed on a medium that contained an adequate concentration of cholesterol.[100] The hatchability of house fly eggs with a normal sterol concentration of 0.96 μg/g did not suffer until the concentration fell to 0.25 μg/g of eggs; at this time the ovipositing females had lost about two thirds of their original body cholesterol.[89] The reported inhibition of hatchability of cotton leafworm eggs by 0.1% sitosterol in the adult diet[54] should be reinvestigated based on the discovery of inhibitors of sterol metabolism in commercial sitosterol.[101]

4. Maturation of Progeny

Adult house flies were held on a diet that contained 0.1% stigmastanol and 0.005% cholesterol, enough sterol for normal hatch (80 to 90%) but not enough to allow larval maturation in the absence of cholesterol. No adults were obtained when the larvae were placed on a 0.2% cholestanol medium, and only 1% of the eggs became adults with 0.005% cholesterol in the larval diet. With 0.2% cholestanol and 0.005% cholesterol in the larval diet, 92% pupation and 61% adult emergence were observed,[40] showing the sparing sterol action of cholestanol and the absolute requirement for some cholesterol.

Ovarian transfer of an essential sterol to progeny was recently demonstrated with axenic *D. melanogaster.*[55] Although cholesterol was not essential for oogenesis, it was required for larval maturation. Flies reared from a cholesterol medium laid viable eggs which matured to adults on media containing either cholesterol or cholestanol. When the cholestanol reared F_1 adults were permitted to lay eggs on the two media, only those ovipositing on cholesterol produced progeny. These females no longer had enough cholesterol left in their bodies to transmit to their eggs to allow F_2 progeny development on diets containing only cholestanol.[55]

5. Male Fertility

Although many studies relating sterols to female insect reproduction have been made, only a few dealt with the male reproductive system. One is discussed later in

Table 4
PERCENT ADULTS FROM EGGS PRODUCED BY INDIVIDUAL MATINGS BETWEEN FLIES REARED FROM THE CHOLESTANOL AND CHOLESTEROL MEDIA[55]

F_1 female dietary sterol	F_1 male dietary sterol	Percent F_2 adults from eggs oviposted on media that contained: Cholesterol	Cholestanol
cholestanol	cholestanol	84	0
cholestanol	cholesterol	87	6
cholesterol	cholestanol	74	78
cholesterol	cholesterol	91	67

the section on ecdysone. In the cholesterol-cholestanol study with *D. melanogaster*, male fertility was not affected by cholestanol or a lack of cholesterol in the medium.[55] Neither was progeny survival on a cholestanol medium affected by the male parent's dietary sterol (Table 4). If any cholesterol was present in the semen, not enough of it entered the egg during ferilization to enable many progeny from cholestanol reared females to mature on a cholestanol medium.

C. Sterols for Defensive Purposes

The metabolism of dietary sterols to progesterone, pregnenolone, and dehydroepiandrosterone was first noted in the confused flour beetle, but no explanation was given for their presence in these insects.[102] In subsequent studies with water beetles, numerous C_{18}, C_{19}, and C_{21} steroids were isolated from their thoracic bladders and were shown to be deleterious to fish and amphibians.[51] The biosynthesis of cardiac glycosides from dietary phytosterols was demonstrated with another group of beetles.[103] The glycosides are excreted from the defensive glands of the insects through pores in the cuticle and render the beetles toxic or unpalatable to predators.

Monarch butterflies and grasshoppers feeding on various milkweed plants, sequester cardiac glycosides from the plants and use them as feeding deterrents against birds.[104,105] In tests with bluejays, butterfly larvae reared on plants containing the glycosides caused vomiting, whereas when the same insects were fed cabbage or other nontoxic plants, they were eaten by the birds without causing vomiting or other ill effects.

In a final example, tomatine, a steroid alkaloid saponin similar to digitonin, is eaten by the corn earworm when feeding on tomato plants. The earworm is unaffected by the compound, but a parasite on the worm, an ichneumenoid wasp, is poisoned by tomatine. The alkaloid interferes with the predator's sterol metabolism.[106]

D. Summary

The function of sterols in insects parallels their function in other animals. They are constituents of biological membranes, and although differences between insects exist, a wide variety of sterol structures appear to be suitable for this role. Sterols are precursors to the arthropod sterol hormones, the ecdysteroids, which control growth, maturation, differentiation, and probably also reproduction in both sexes. Sterols and their esters are placed by female insects into their eggs just as cholesterol is deposited by the hen into her eggs, to provide a source of this compound necessary for embryogenesis. And sterols are used by some insects, just as they are used by some animals, for defensive secretions and to render themselves unpalatable or toxic to predators.

Inability to synthesize sterols does not inhibit their use by insects. Since these compounds are so prevalent among all living organisms, it is hard to imagine a natural insect food that doesn't contain them. There is no known instance where a sterol deficiency in an insects' normal diet is a limiting factor for growth and reproduction. In those cases where dietary sterol levels are very low, as in the plant sap taken up by aphids or in the wood eaten by termites, symbiotic microorganisms in the insects' intestinal tracts probably furnish their hosts adequate sterols. To date, most insects cannot be reared away from their natural diet or in the absence of microorganisms.

V. METABOLISM

An early study of the metabolism of sterols by insects used paper chromatography to show that the major tissue sterol in the confused flour beetle was 7-dehydrocholesterol even though cholesterol, cholestanol, sitosterol, or ergosterol were the dietary sterols.[39] Two years later, Clark and Bloch[7] isolated ^{14}C-22-dehydrocholesterol from German cockroaches that had been fed ^{14}C-ergosterol in their diet. These demonstrations of dealkylation and selective double bond introduction or saturation initiated extensive studies on sterol metabolism by insects.

A. Hydrolysis, Esterification, and Conjugation

1. Hydrolysis

The hydrolysis of dietary sterol esters can be inferred from the many nutritional studies in which cholesteryl acetate and other cholesteryl esters were used as readily as cholesterol by insects (Table 1). In a specific study with a roach,[78] cholesteryl acetate, laurate, palmitate, stearate, and oleate were all hydrolyzed to cholesterol by the insect. The esters could be absorbed through the gut without prior hydrolysis, and appeared to be taken up more readily by crop and carcass tissues than free cholesterol. No comparable studies with sterol glycosides or acyl sterol glycosides have yet been done.

2. Esterification

Esters of dietary cholesterol were found in 17 separate tissues and organs of the American cockroach and represented 48% of the total sterols in the hemolymph and salivary glands.[83] Cholesterol, 7-dehydrocholesterol, and lathosterol were all esterified by homogenates of gut tissue, whereas coprostanol, sitosterol, stigmasterol, and ergosterol were not.[83] In a later study, 29% of the carcass cholesterol was esterified after the cockroaches were fed ^{14}C-cholesterol in their diet for 60 days. Assay for radioactivity demonstrated that free cholesterol does not readily equilibrate with its esters in the insects.[27]

Sterol esters comprised 41% of the total sterols in house fly eggs but only 8.4% of the sterols in adults. Over 90% of the esters were palmitoleate and oleate.[90] Esterification of dietary cholesterol was minimal during the growth of house fly larvae; it increased during pupation and adulthood.[89] The low concentration of sterol esters in house fly larvae was recently confirmed. Only 1% of dietary ^{14}C-cholesterol occurred as esters in the larvae, and this low percentage remained invariant as the dietary cholesterol concentration was increased from 0.02 to 22 mg per gram of diet.[16]

In an extensive series of investigations with the cockroach, Clayton and co-workers showed that 6 hr after ingestion of dietary ^{14}C-cholesterol, 28% of it was present as esters in the crop while almost none was esterified in the hemolymph (blood).[78] Cholesteryl oleate was the predominant ester synthesized by the cockroaches on dietary regimens containing three different fatty acid mixtures.[107] When the insects were reared on a diet containing subminimal quantities (0.005%) of ^{14}C-cholesterol and larger amounts (0.1%) of ^{3}H-cholestanol as a sparing sterol, the latter was converted to esters in varying degrees depending on the tissue, leaving the cholesterol almost entirely in the metabolically active "free" state. Highest concentrations of sterol esters were in the intestinal tract, fat body, and nerve tissues.[23,79] Part of the cholestanol was desaturated to lathosterol, which was also esterified and stored in the fat of the growing insects.[79]

In the neutral lipids of large termites, cholesterol esters predominated over free cholesterol in the fat body, heads, thoraces, and abdomens of females. They were relatively low (17% of total sterols) in large soldier termites and high (75% of total sterols) in the winged, sexually mature reproductive castes.[86] In the Mexican bean beetle, 29 to 38% of the tissue sterols were esterified when either labeled cholestanol, cholesterol, stigmastanol, stigmasterol, or sitosterol were administered with the diet.[95] The milkweed bug, which incorporated dietary sterols (campesterol, stigmasterol, sitosterol) into its tissues without appreciable structural modification, esterified all of them to the extent of 65% (adult males), 47% (adult females), and 11% (eggs) of the total sterol fraction in these three forms.[80] In a primitive insect, the silverfish, a large proportion of the carcass sterols were esterified. Although only 8% of the body weight was lipid, 20 to 25% of this fraction was sterol esters and only 4 to 5% free sterols.[87]

Sterol esters were not detected in the hemolymph of the cricket[85] and were absent in the hemolymph of the cockroach.[78] Their presence in the hemolymph of the American cockroach (48% of total sterols)[83] renders their status in insect blood ambiguous. They may play no significant role in sterol transport in some insects[85] yet be important, as in mammals, for transport in others. More research is required to clarify this point. Finally, the increase is sterol ester in the lipids of maturing silkworm ovaries correlates with the high requirement for these compounds in the eggs.[88]

3. Conjugation

The conjugation of dietary sterols for excretion was investigated with only one insect. The meconium (intestinal contents eliminated during pupal-adult molt) of the tobacco hornworm was shown to contain the sulfates of cholesterol, campesterol, and sitosterol.[108] Conjugation and excretion of ecdysteroids has been investigated more frequently and will be discussed in a later section.

B. Introduction of Double Bonds

1. Desaturation of Cholesterol to 7-Dehydrocholesterol

The conversion of dietary cholesterol to 7-dehydrocholesterol by the confused flour beetle was the first demonstration of desaturation of sterols by insects.[39] This metabolic step is the reverse of one of the last stages of cholesterol biosynthesis in mammals and was shown *not* to occur in guinea pigs.[109] The desaturation was substantiated with labeled cholesterol and axenic colonies of German cockroaches,[98] and house flies.[89] House flies, unable to use sitosterol except as a sparing sterol, also convert it in part to 7-dehydrositosterol.[110]

HO H LATHOSTEROL —MAMMALS→ HO 7-DEHYDRO-CHOLESTEROL —MAMMALS→ / ←INSECTS— HO CHOLESTEROL

The stereochemistry of the desaturation was established with 7α and 7β-tritiated 4-^{14}C-cholesterol and a blow fly. The 7β and 8β hydrogen atoms were removed in the insect by an enzymatic *cis*-dehydrogenation step.[36]

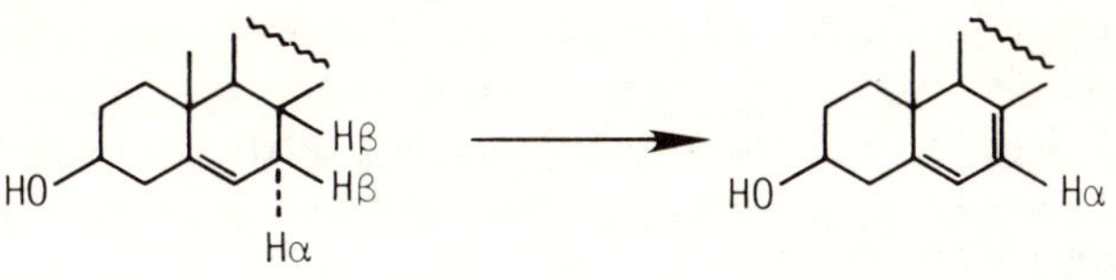

CHOLESTEROL → 7-DEHYDROCHOLESTEROL

Not all insects, however, can desaturate cholesterol to 7-dehydrocholesterol. *D. pachea*[48] and the ambrosia beetle[47] were able to complete their life cycles with 7-dehydrocholesterol but not cholesterol in their diets. In contrast, two locust species[21] and the pales weevil[35] were reported to use cholesterol, but not 7-dehydrocholesterol as a dietary sterol. Two others, a flesh fly[31] and the oriental house fly[15] used the latter sterol less effectively than cholesterol.

2. Desaturation of Cholestanol

In the earliest investigation (1961), it was shown that labeled cholestanol was not converted to cholesterol by a cockroach.[23] During the next year, the German cockroach was shown to convert dietary cholestanol into lathosterol[68,98] and this conversion was subsequently demonstrated in another cockroach,[111] house fly,[98] and blow fly.[36] In an investigation with suitably labeled cholestanols, loss of the 7β and 8β hydrogen atoms was shown to occur.[111] The 7α and 7β-hydroxycholestanols were not intermediates in the reaction.

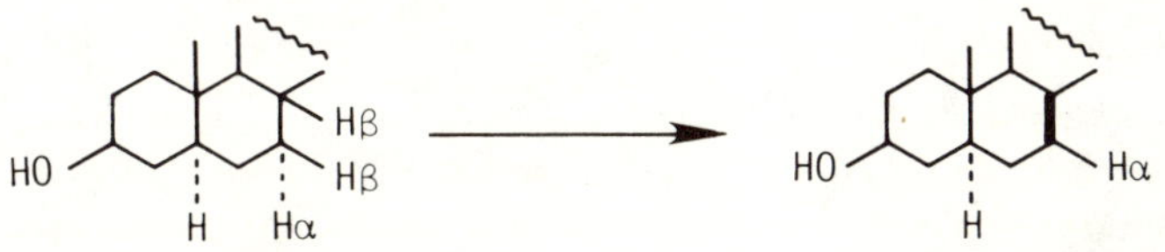

CHOLESTANOL → LATHOSTEROL

Desaturation of cholestanol to lathosterol does not occur in *D. pachea.* The insect, which requires a Δ^7-sterol in its diet, dies during its early larval stages on a diet containing only cholestanol.[56] Cholestanol and lathosterol were separately tested as dietary sterols with only one insect, *D. melanogaster.*[37] Both were rated as "less effective" than cholesterol for larval growth. The metabolism of cholestanol has never been investigated with an insect that could use it as the sole dietary sterol.

3. Desaturation of Other Sterols

Removal of the C_{24} and C_{28} hydrogen atoms from phytosterols by insects is discussed later in the section dealing with dealkylation.

Desaturation of lathosterol to 7-dehydrocholesterol occurred in axenic cultures of *D. pachea,*[76] an insect which lacks the ability to convert Δ^5-sterols to $\Delta^{5,7}$-derivatives. In the only other instance investigated, the metabolism of lathosterol to 7-dehydrocholesterol was *not* observed in the blow fly.[36]

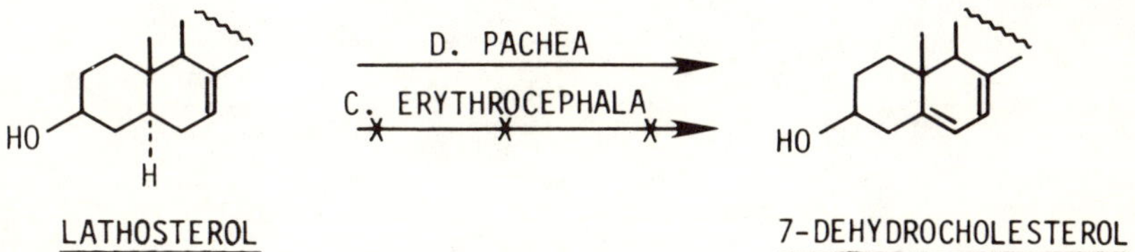

LATHOSTEROL → (D. PACHEA; not C. ERYTHROCEPHALA) → 7-DEHYDROCHOLESTEROL

The formation of defensive secretions by dysticid water beetles requires a truncation of the sterol side chain and introduction of a $\Delta^{4,6}$-3-ketone system.[51] When suitably labeled cholesterol derivatives were injected into one of the species of this group, loss of the 4α and 7β hydrogen atoms occurred during the conversion of cholesterol to the $\Delta^{4,6}$-3-ketopregnadienes.[112]

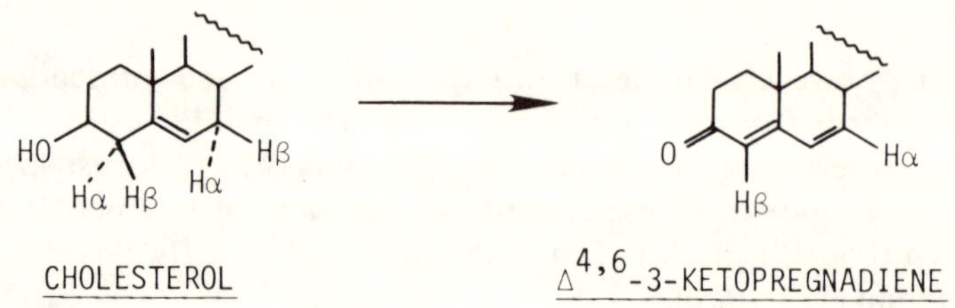

HO Hα Hβ Hα Hβ → O Hβ Hα

CHOLESTEROL → $\Delta^{4,6}$-3-KETOPREGNADIENE

C. Saturation of Double Bonds

1. $\Delta^{5,7}$ to Δ^{5}-Sterols

Metabolism of ergosterol to 22-dehydrocholesterol by the German cockroach was the first example of double bond reduction in a sterol by an insect.[7] A comparable reduction of 7-dehydrocholesterol to cholesterol by the confused flour beetle was later reported in a review which also stated that a $\Delta^{5,7}$-diene system was probably necessary for saturation of the Δ^{7}-double bond in insects.[51]

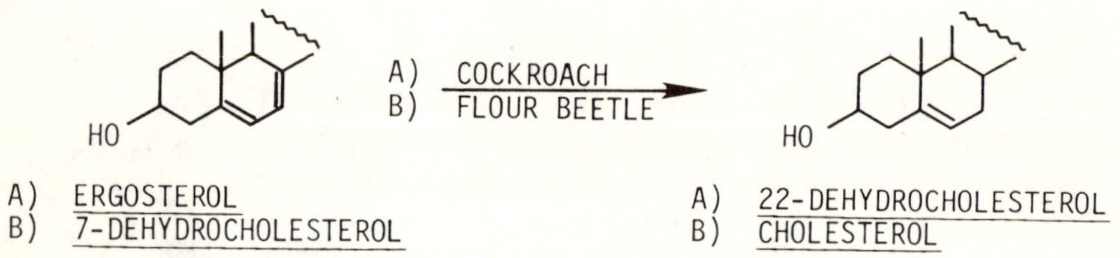

HO — A) COCKROACH / B) FLOUR BEETLE → HO

A) ERGOSTEROL
B) 7-DEHYDROCHOLESTEROL

A) 22-DEHYDROCHOLESTEROL
B) CHOLESTEROL

2. Desmosterol ($\Delta^{5,24}$) to Cholesterol (Δ^{5})

The principal work in this area was carried out with the tobacco hornworm, an insect that effectively dealkylates a number of common phytosterols to cholesterol.[52] Desmosterol occurs as an intermediate during the dealkylation[59] and is normally reduced to cholesterol with NADPH and a reductase associated with the microsomal fraction in the midgut of the insect.[113]

A considerable literature exists on inhibitors of this reduction. Triparanol (MER-29) and 22,25-diazacholesterol specifically block Δ^{24} saturation of desmosterol to cholesterol in vertebrates and also inhibit this reduction in the tobacco hornworm with severe retardation of larval growth.[29] Incorporation of 20,25-diazacholesterol together with a number of phytosterols into the diet of the hornworm caused an accumulation of desmosterol in its tissues in every case.[52] An impurity found in commercial sitosterol, 3β-hydroxy-24-norchol-5-en-23-oic acid, also caused a buildup of desmosterol in the insect but had no deleterious effects on the growth and development of the hornworm larvae.[101] The acid was shown to be an inhibitor of the Δ^{24}-reductase in both rats and insects.[113]

Table 5
INHIBITION OF Δ²⁴-SATURATION IN INSECTS WITH 20,25-DIAZACHOLESTEROL[114]

Insect	% of total sterols		
	Cholesterol	Desmosterol	Sitosterol
Tobacco hornworm larvae	5.6	21.8	72.6
Corn earworm larvae	1.0	18.6	80.4
Fall armyworm larvae	2.8	34.9	52.3
Firebrat nymphs	69.8	11.4	17.8
German cockroach nymphs	47.3	33.2	19.5
American cockroach nymphs	30.9	16.5	52.6
American cockroach adult males	83.0	4.0	13.0
American cockroach adult females	49.7	6.1	44.2
Control, all insects, no diazasterol	80-90	<2	10-20

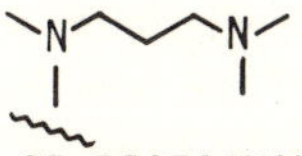

20,25-DIAZACHOLESTEROL

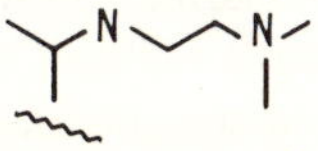

22,25-DIAZACHOLESTEROL

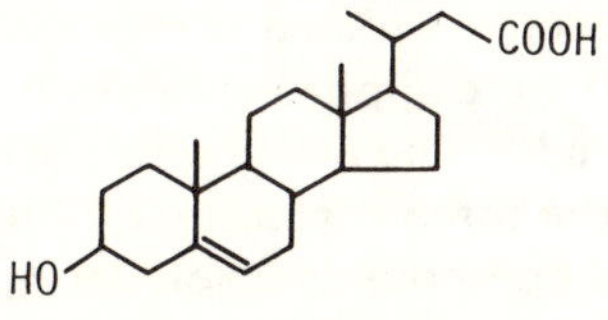

3β-HYDROXY-24-NORCHOL-5-EN-23-OIC ACID

Not all insects respond equally to Δ^{24}-reductase inhibitors. In an extensive survey with numerous azasterols and various insects, inclusion of 0.2% 20,25-diazacholesterol in diets containing 0.2% sitosterol resulted in the following sterol composition in the insects. (Table 5)

In an independent study with three species of cockroaches, the dealkylation of sitosterol to cholesterol was also not seriously inhibited by azasterols or the norcholenic acid.[115] Triparanol prevented the saturation of desmosterol to cholesterol during the dealkylation of clionasterol in the yellow mealworm and allowed desmosterol to be isolated from the insect.[116]

3. 22-Dehydrodesmosterol to Cholesterol

Reduction of the Δ^{22} bond precedes that of the Δ^{24} bond during dealkylation of stigmasterol by the tobacco hornworm. Little, if any, conversion of 22-dehydrocholesterol to cholesterol takes place in this insect.[117]

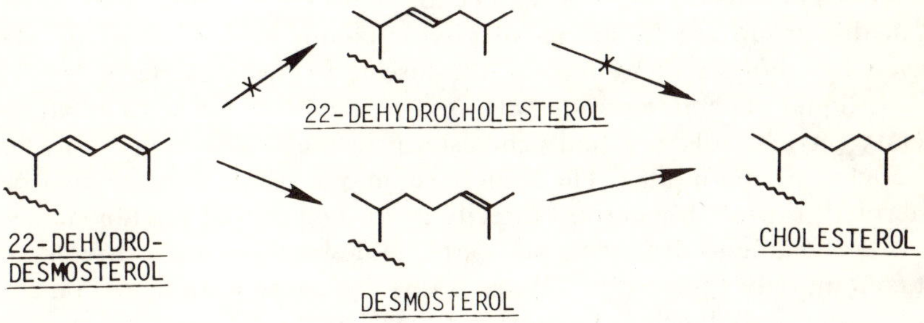

22-DEHYDROCHOLESTEROL

22-DEHYDRO-DESMOSTEROL

CHOLESTEROL

DESMOSTEROL

4. Cholestanone to Cholestanol

The discovery that cholestanone but not Δ^4-cholesten-3-one was a sparing sterol for cholesterol in the diet of house flies suggested that the saturated ketone was reduced to a stanol by the insects. When ^{14}C-cholestanone was incorporated into larval diets together with subminimal amounts of cholesterol, ^{14}C-cholestanol was iosolated from the pupae. This was the first clearcut example of the reduction of a carbonyl group to an alcohol by insects.[40]

5. The Mexican Bean Beetle, a Special Case

Analysis of host plant and carcass sterols indicated an unusual example of insect sterol metabolism in the Mexican bean beetle.[94] The sterols in the soybean leaves upon which the insect fed consisted principally of campesterol (11%), stigmasterol (31.5%), and sitosterol (55%), whereas the sterols in adult beetles were cholesterol (4.5%), cholestanol (50.7%), lathosterol (11.8%), campestanol (6%), and stigmastanol (20.3%). Saturated sterols comprised only 1.4% of the total in the leaves, but 77% of those in the insect. Of the remaining 33% unsaturated sterols in the Mexican bean beetle, about half were Δ^7 sterols.

In a subsequent study, tritiated sterols (cholestanol, cholesterol, stigmastanol, stigmasterol, sitosterol) were applied to soybean leaves and the fate of the compounds in the insects determined.[95] The two cholestane derivatives were assimilated by the insects more readily than the three stigmastanes, but all were partially esterified (30 to 40%) and the unsaturated compounds (cholesterol, stigmasterol, sitosterol) reduced to stanols (52 to 77%). Only traces of cholestanol and 1.3% of the labeled stigmastanol were desaturated to Δ^7-sterols. Over 50% of the unsaturated sterol fraction derived from cholesterol was lathosterol, and dealkylation of stigmasterol and sitosterol but not stigmastanol occurred. In an extension of this study, the predacious *Coccinella septempunctata*, a relative of the Mexican bean beetle that feeds on aphids, does not convert dietary sterols to stanols.[95a]

In conclusion, the Mexican bean beetle reduces dietary Δ^5 sterols to stanols, dealkylates C_{29} sterols to C_{27} derivatives and probably synthesizes Δ^7-sterols from Δ^5-sterols via the $\Delta^{5,7}$-dienes rather than from stanols as has been previously observed.[68,111]

D. Dealkylation at C-24 in the Phytosterol Side Chain

1. Removal of the C_{24}-Ethyl Group

The dealkylation of sitosterol to cholesterol was also first demonstrated with the omnivorous German cockroach.[118] Insects fed 0.2% ^{3}H-sitosterol in the diet for 42 days were worked up for sterols to yield 80% ^{3}H-cholesterol and 6% unchanged sitosterol. Similar results were subsequently obtained with the Virginia pine sawfly,[119] tobacco hornworm,[59] confused flour beetle,[59] silkworm,[120] honey bee,[121] and three cockroaches.[115] The dealkylation was also inferred in numerous instances when sitosterol was the principal or only dietary sterol and cholesterol the principal insect tissue sterol. Included in this group are 16 species of phytophagous insects reared on plants and then assayed for cholesterol by feeding the insects to the cholesterol requiring hide beetle.[43] Gas-liquid chromatography was used to establish the same relationship between dietary phytosterols and body cholesterol in the boll weevil,[50] grasshopper,[122] termite,[86] cricket,[123] and moth.[93] The cholesterol in queens of the oriental hornet (95% of total sterols)[84] is probably derived directly from their diet of phytophagous insects. Five insects are unable to dealkylate sitosterol. Hide beetle nymphs do not survive on diets that contain only sitosterol.[6,43] When house fly larvae were reared on a diet containing 0.1% randomly labeled ^{3}H-sitosterol, 99% of the ^{3}H-sterols in the pupae was sitosterol.[28,110] Analysis of the milkweed bug and the sunflower seeds on which it feeds shows that little, if any, conversion of C_{28} and C_{29} dietary sterols to cholesterol occurred.[80] Labeled campesterol, sitosterol and 24-methylenecholesterol were fed to honey bee workers in chemically defined diets and the sterols of prepapae and newly emerged queens which had been fed by the workers were analyzed. None of the three sterols were dealkylated and there was no conversion of the first two to the third.[80a] Also neither labeled sitosterol, stigmasterol or desmosterol were converted to cholesterol when fed to or injected into the Khapra beetle.[80b]

The first detection of an intermediate in the dealkylation of sitosterol was the isolation of ^{3}H-desmosterol when ^{3}H-sitosterol was placed in the diet of the tobacco hornworm.[59] No significant conversion of ^{14}C-cholesterol could be detected in the insect. The second intermediate established in the dealkylation of sitosterol was fucosterol.[124,125] During the same year (1971), Japanese workers demonstrated the chemical conversion of fucosterol 24,28-epoxide to desmosterol with boron trifluoride etherate and suggested a similar reaction might be the basis of phytosterol dealkylation in insects.[126] They also noted that 24-methylene-cholesterol epoxide gave no detectable desmosterol under the same conditions.

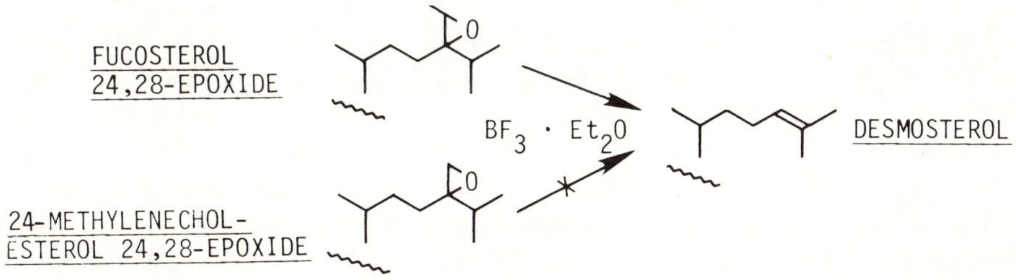

FUCOSTEROL 24,28-EPOXIDE

$BF_3 \cdot Et_2O$

DESMOSTEROL

24-METHYLENECHOLESTEROL 24,28-EPOXIDE

As a test, silkworm larvae were injected with ^{3}H-fucosterol epoxide and the sterols isolated from them 1 hr later; 15% incorporation of ^{3}H into cholesterol had occurred. The following mechanism was proposed:[24]

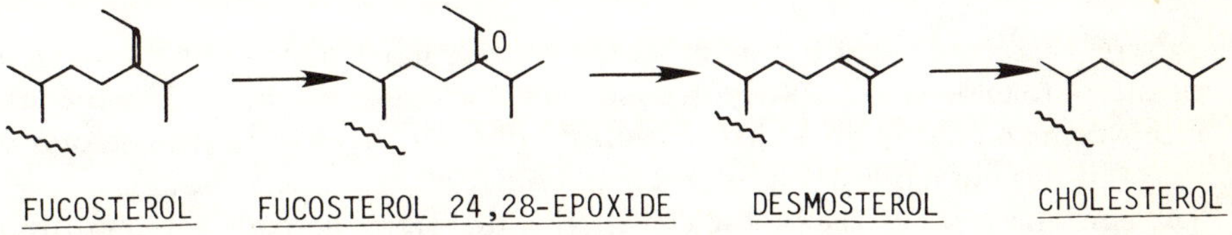

FUCOSTEROL → FUCOSTEROL 24,28-EPOXIDE → DESMOSTEROL → CHOLESTEROL

These results were confirmed the following year with locusts. After injection of ^{3}H-fucosterol epoxide into the abdomen of mature larvae, all of the radioactivity was found in the cholesterol and none in the campestane or stigmastane derivatives isolated from the insects.[127] Four additional aspects of the dealkylation mechanism were recently worked out.

1. The retention of the C_{25} hydrogen atom was observed during the dealkylations of isofucosterol to cholesterol,[128] clionasterol to desmosterol[117,129] and 24ξ-ethylcholesterol to desmosterol[130] which led the investigators to propose the following steps:

O ENZYME　　O⁻ ENZYME

25-^{3}H-FUCOSTEROL 24,28-EPOXIDE　　ENZYME LINKED INTERMEDIATES　　24-^{3}H-DESMOSTEROL

2. Oxygenated intermediates during the dealkylation other than fucosterol epoxide were not found, nor would the following derivatives substitute as effective dietary sterols for the silkworm:[41]

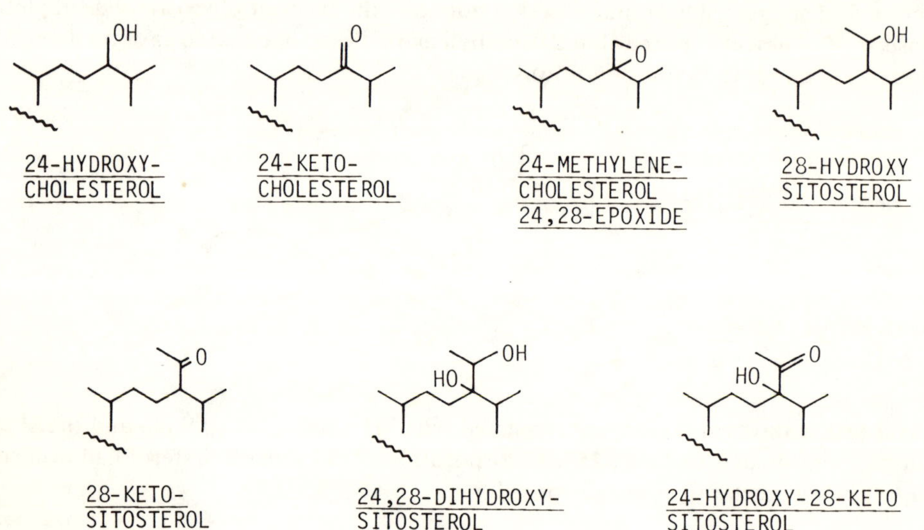

and are therefore ruled out as probable intermediates during the conversion of sitosterol to cholesterol. 28-Hydroxysitosterol was also not utilized by the yellow mealworm and although 24-hydroxysitosterol was converted to fucosterol by this insect, it was not a normal sitosterol metabolite.[41a]

3. The configuration of the biologically active fucosterol epoxide was shown to be 24S,25S by preparation of the two possible isomers. The two were tritiated and incorporated into gut homogenates from silkworm larvae. Only the 24S,25S isomer was transformed into desmosterol.[131] More recent work however, showed that both isomers of fucosterol 24,28-epoxide are formed in the silkworm gut[131a] and are converted to cholesterol by this tissue.[131b] In addition, although both isomers of isofucosterol epoxide were converted to cholesterol by the yellow mealworm, the (24R,28S)-epoxide was converted 10 times as much as the (24S,28R) isomer.[131c] Neither isomer of isofucosterol epoxide was converted to cholesterol by the silkworm[131b] even though both fucosterol and isofucosterol were detected by GC-MS in this insect.[131d]

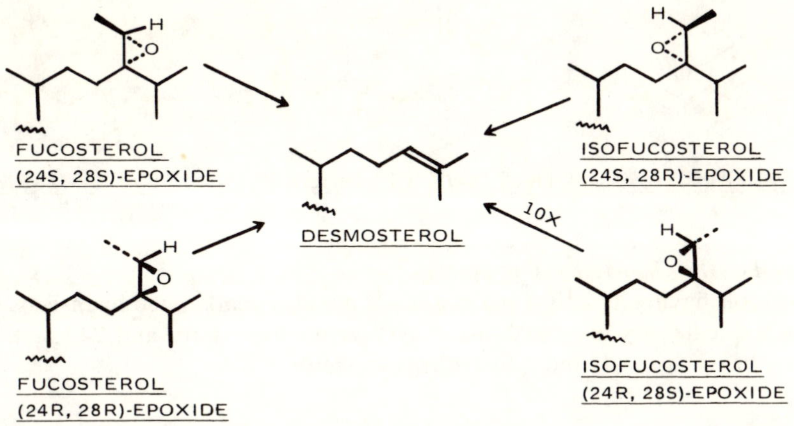

FUCOSTEROL
(24S, 28S)-EPOXIDE

ISOFUCOSTEROL
(24S, 28R)-EPOXIDE

DESMOSTEROL

10X

FUCOSTEROL
(24R, 28R)-EPOXIDE

ISOFUCOSTEROL
(24R, 28S)-EPOXIDE

4. Removal of the 24α-ethyl group of stigmasterol and reduction of the Δ^{22}-*trans* double bond was shown to go via 22-dehydrodesmosterol and desmosterol in the tobacco hornworm.[117] Very little, if any, conversion of *trans*-22-dehydrocholesterol to cholesterol occurred in this insect.

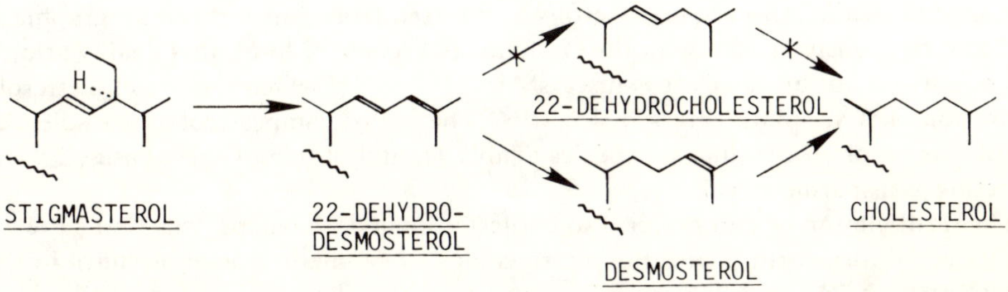

STIGMASTEROL

22-DEHYDRO-
DESMOSTEROL

22-DEHYDROCHOLESTEROL

DESMOSTEROL

CHOLESTEROL

The dealkylation of stigmasterol to cholesterol can now be represented by the following sequence (sitosterol would be the same, without the Δ^{22}-unsaturation):

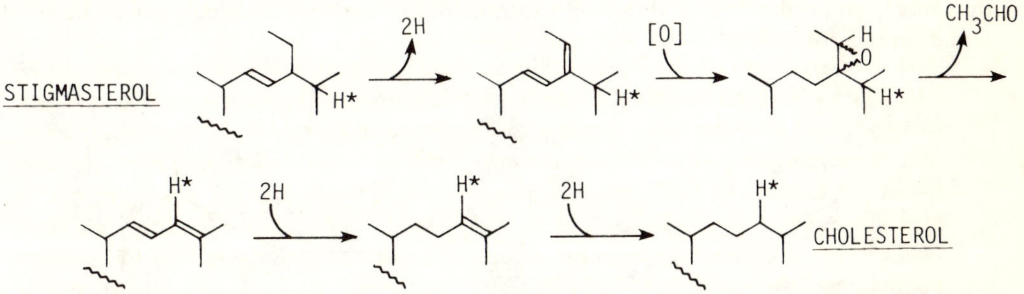

STIGMASTEROL

2H

[O]

CH_3CHO

H*

CHOLESTEROL

Several dealkylation inhibitors have been prepared. 24,28-Iminofucosterol, a general toxin to the silkworm,[63] specifically inhibited the fucosterol → desmosterol step.[132] Of the two allenic sterols, cholesta-5,23,24-trien-3β-ol was also a general toxin but did not affect dealkylation, whereas stigmasta-5,24(28),28-trien-3β-ol was nontoxic but inhibited the conversions of sitosterol to fucosterol and of the latter to its epoxide.[133]

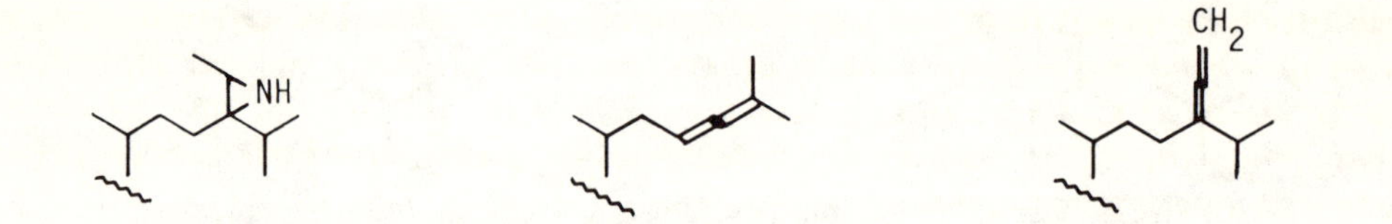

NH CH$_2$

24,28-IMINOFUCOSTEROL CHOLESTA-5,23 24-TRIEN-3β-OL STIGMASTA-5,24(28), 28-TRIEN-3β-OL

2. Removal of the C_{24}-Methyl Group

Phytosterols having a methyl group at C-24 are also dealkylated by insects. Common sterols in this category are the 24α-methyl sterol campesterol and 24β-methyl sterols ergosterol, brassicasterol, and dihydrobrassicasterol.

H CH$_3$ CH$_3$ H CH$_3$ H

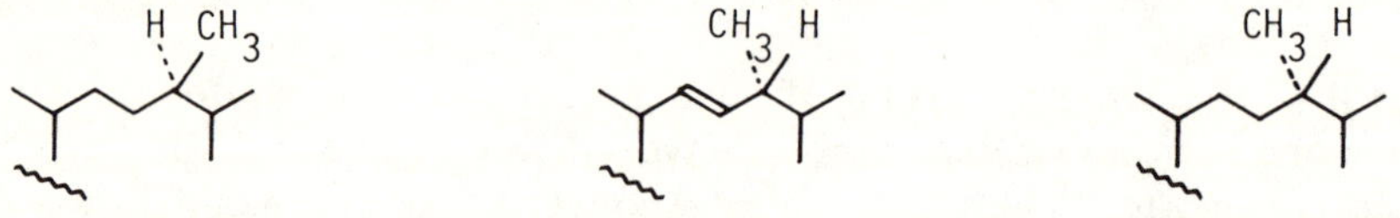

CAMPESTEROL ERGOSTEROL, BRASSICASTEROL DIHYDROBRASSICASTEROL

The specific dealkylation of ergosterol was inferred from paper chromatographic studies[39] and rigorously proved with the German cockroach.[7] 24β-Methyl dealkylation cannot be carried out by carnivorus insects[1,6,19,22,25,31,42,43,57] which require cholesterol and even some that are plant eaters.[21,33,35,38,44,48] The use of campesterol as the sole dietary sterol was reported for only six species (Table 1), and in one of these cases,[42,57] it may be acting as a sparing sterol.

The dealkylation of campesterol to cholesterol via desmosterol was first shown with the tobacco hornworm,[52] and the intermediacy of 24-methylene-cholesterol in the removal of both 24α and 24β-methyl groups was also demonstrated with this insect.[58] However, where fucosterol 24,28-epoxide is an intermediate in the conversion of fucosterol to desmosterol, the comparable 24-methylenecholesterol epoxide is not converted to desmosterol either by BF_3-etherate[126] or the silkworm.[41] The mechanism by which the 24-methylene group is removed by insects is still unknown. The pathway that has been established to date lacks intermediates between 24-methylenecholesterol and desmosterol:

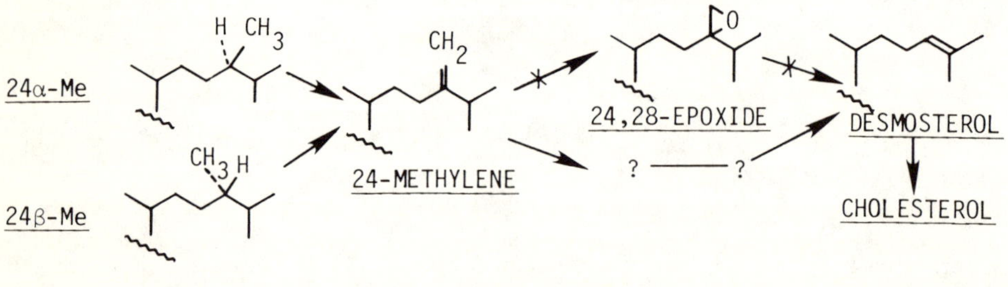

H CH$_3$ CH$_2$ O

24α-Me 24,28-EPOXIDE DESMOSTEROL

CH$_3$ H ? —— ?

24β-Me 24-METHYLENE CHOLESTEROL

At least one phytophagous insect does not dealkylate campesterol. The milkweed bug not only incorporates this dietary sterol into its tissues unchanged,[80] but also synthesizes an ecdysteroid from campesterol without prior removal of the 24α-methyl group.[134]

E. Truncations and Removal of the Side Chain

The metabolism of ingested sterols to other steroids takes place in numerous insects. In the earliest investigation,[102] confused flour beetle larvae were reared from egg to maturity on a diet of flour and yeast (ergosterol). After extraction, saponification and workup, dehydroepiandrosterone, pregnenolone, and progesterone were identified in the larvae by TLC, GLC, and physical constants of the ketones and their 2,4-dinitrophenylhydrazones. The authors concluded that side chain splitting enzymes are present in insects as well as mammals.

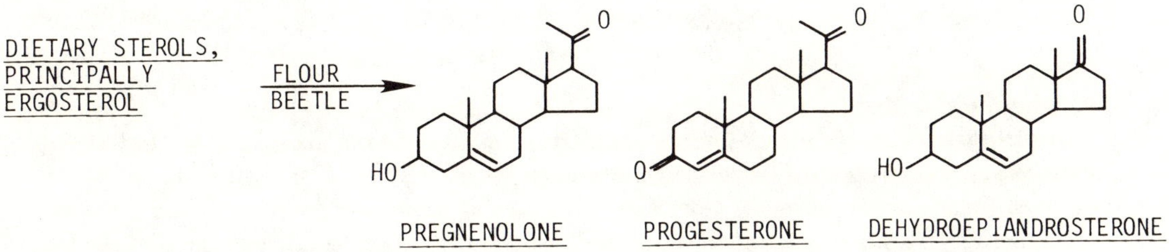

DIETARY STEROLS, PRINCIPALLY ERGOSTEROL — FLOUR BEETLE → PREGNENOLONE, PROGESTERONE, DEHYDROEPIANDROSTERONE

In a series of papers, Schildknecht and co-workers (review[51]) isolated numerous C_{18}, C_{19}, and C_{21} steroids (e.g., cybisterol) from thoracic bladders of water beetles. The steroids, used as defensive substances by the beetles, were synthesized from injected cholesterol and progesterone by the insects, but not from mevalonolactone.

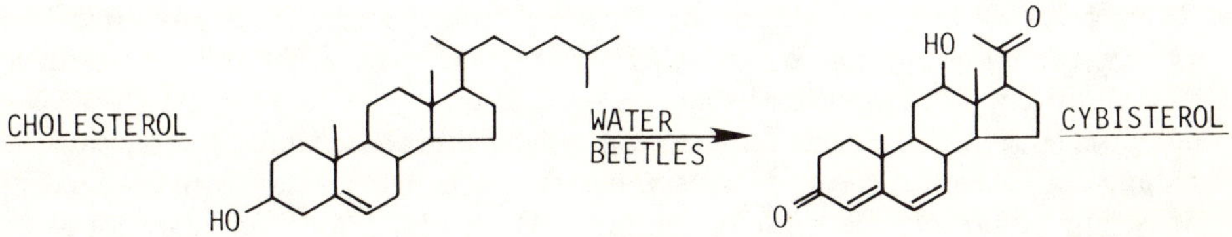

CHOLESTEROL — WATER BEETLES → CYBISTEROL

In another example, cardiac glycosides were identified in the defensive secretions of chrysomelid beetles (9 of 20 species in 3 genera).[103] The glycosides were absent from the host plants upon which the insects were reared, and were synthesized from ingested sterols. Exact structures of the aglycones were not determined, but the sugars were reported to be arabinose and xylose.

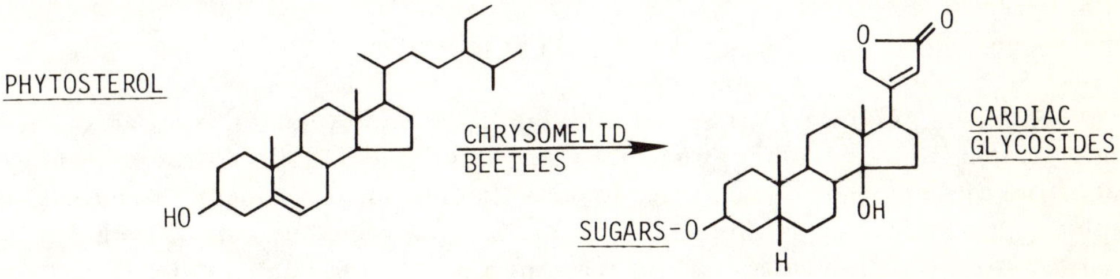

PHYTOSTEROL — CHRYSOMELID BEETLES → CARDIAC GLYCOSIDES

This extensive metabolic process probably involves conversion of the dietary sterol to a progesterone derivative followed by reductions, hydroxylations, conjugation with pentoses and condensation with a 2-carbon substrate to form the butenolide ring.

Another drastic removal of a sterol side chain and rebuilding is suggested by the recent isolation of 4 bufadienolides from fireflies.[135] This is the first time such compounds were found in insects.

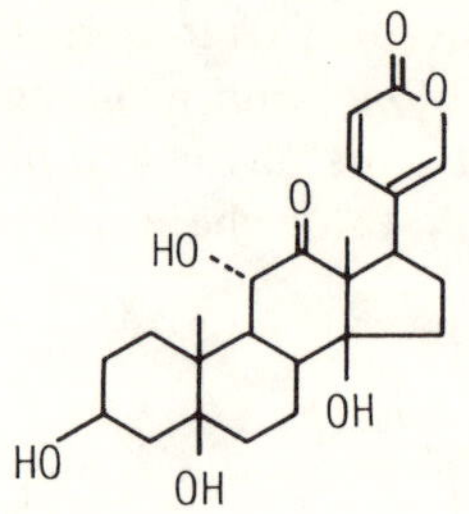

FIREFLY BUFALIN

F. Summary

Hydrolysis of sterol esters and esterification of free sterols are common, but varies between species as well as sexes, ages, and tissues of insects. Concentrations of sterol esters appear higher in eggs, where they may exist as a storage form ready for easy mobilization during embryogenesis. A selective uptake of sterols from the diet probably occurs in most insects and these compounds are selectively deposited in various tissues.

Most phytophagous insects are able to remove the methyl and ethyl groups at C_{24} in plant sterols and convert them to cholesterol. All carnivorous and some omnivorous species seem to lack this ability and require some cholesterol in their diets for maturation and reproduction. The intermediacy of fucosterol, fucosterol 24,28-epoxide, and desmosterol during the dealkylation of sitosterol to cholesterol is firmly established, but no oxygenated intermediate between 24-methylene cholesterol and desmosterol in the dealkylation of 24-methyl sterols has yet been found.

Some insects are able to remove part or all of the side chain to form progestane and androstane derivatives and even to biosynthesize cardiac glycosides from ingested sterols. Most appear to be able to dehydrogenate Δ^5 sterols to $\Delta^{5,7}$ derivatives and some can convert cholestanol to lathosterol ($\Delta^0 \rightarrow \Delta^7$). Saturation of double bonds also occurs, notably the reduction of desmosterol to cholesterol ($\Delta^{5,24} \rightarrow \Delta^5$). In a special case, an insect converted almost all of its dietary sterols to stanols ($\Delta^5 \rightarrow \Delta^0$). Exceptions to these generalizations occur. The huge numbers of insect species together with their manifold niches in nature are sure to be reflected by significant variations in sterol metabolism. From all of the work done so far, however, exceptions are not the rule, and a foundation for understanding the insect-sterol relationship is gradually forming.

VI. ECDYSONE

Development of insects from egg to adult takes place in several discrete stages. These are separated from each other by a process called molting or *ecdysis.* Groups of insects vary from those in which little change in general appearance is evident throughout life (aphids, grasshoppers, cockroaches) to those exhibiting striking morphological changes from larva or caterpillar through the pupa to the adult (house flies, bees, butterflies).[136] All species must periodically soften (or discard) the old cuticle and synthesize a new one, as this hard exoskeleton would otherwise inhibit growth. A fruit fly larva, for instance, increases in volume about 1000-fold in 8 days during which time there are three ecdyses.

The first demonstration that this process is controlled by hormones that are species nonspecific was made by Kopec in 1922. Hemolymph taken from one insect at the proper time, when injected into those of a different species, caused molting in the latter even though they were not ready for the process.[137] Subsequent experiments by others with organ removal, larval ligations, and tissue reimplantations showed that the hormones controlling ecdysis are synthesized in the brain and in two glands in or directly behind the head of the insect, the corpus allatum and the prothoracic gland.

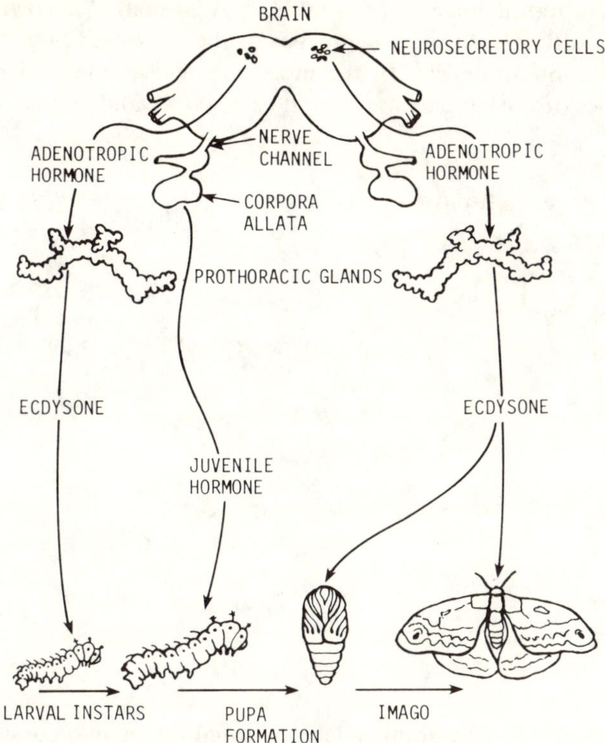

FIGURE 1. Hormonal control of insect growth and metamorphoses.

It is currently believed that neurosecretory cells in the brain respond to a stimulus (temperature, photoperiod, nutritional status, etc.) and make a peptide hormone which in turn travels via nerve axons and the hemolymph to the other glands where it stimulates the corpus allatum to synthesize juvenile hormone and the prothoracic gland to make ecdysone. These two hormones are transported by the hemolymph to their target tissues where they stimulate protein synthesis and induce molting at appropriate times during the maturation of the insect. When acting together, the two hormones cause molting from one immature stage to another; when ecdysone acts alone, the insect changes to the adult, reproductive form [9,138,139] (Figure 1).

A. Structure

In 1954, Butenandt and Karlson[140] isolated 25 mg crystalline ecdysone from 500 kg silkworm pupae. The elemental composition, $C_{27}H_{44}O_6$, suggested a highly oxygenated cholesterol, a premise that was substantiated in 1963 when ^{14}C-cholesterol was shown to be a precursor of the hormone in a blow fly.[8] After an extensive series of investigations[141] the structure of ecdysone was established to be (22R)-2β,3β,14,22,25-pentahydroxy-5β-cholest-7-en-6-one and it was independently synthesized by two groups soon thereafter.[142,143] The juvenile hormone, an epoxy, branched chain, diunsaturated fatty acid methyl ester, was synthesized the following year.[144]

A second ecdysteroid, variously called β-ecdysone, crustecdysone or ecdysterone, was first isolated from a crayfish and shown to be 20-hydroxy-ecdysone.[145] It is now considered to be the principal insect ecdysteroid.[51] Several other ecdysteroids were isolated from insects. 26-Hydroxyecdysone (26.5 mg) was the major hormone in eggs (5 kg) of the tobacco hornworm; ecdysone, 20-hydroxyecdysone, and 20,26-dihydroxyecdysone were present in much smaller amounts.[146] A 24-methyl derivative, Makisterone A, was the main molting hormone in embryos of the milkweed bug,[134] an insect which does not dealkylate plant sterols. In the most recent example, 2-deoxyecdysone was found in the ovaries of the silkworm, where it existed free and as a conjugate in roughly equal quantities.[147]

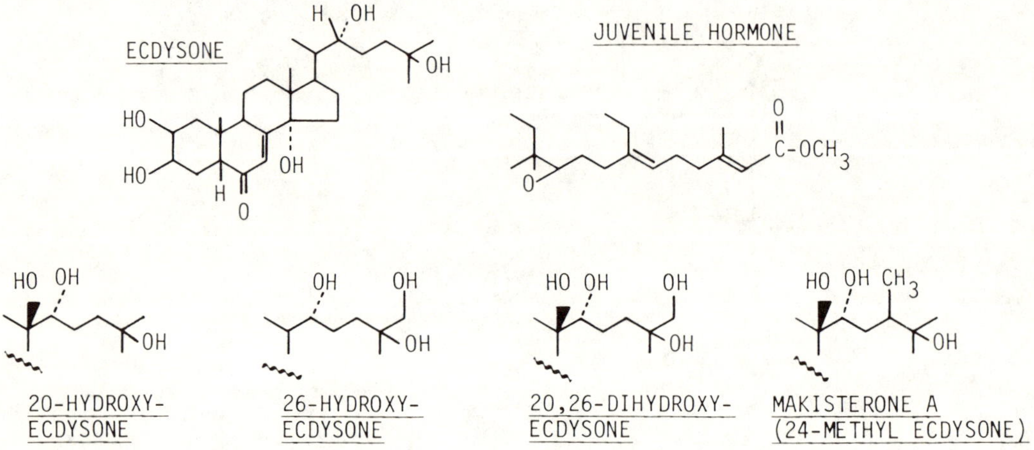

ECDYSONE

JUVENILE HORMONE

20-HYDROXY-ECDYSONE

26-HYDROXY-ECDYSONE

20,26-DIHYDROXY-ECDYSONE

MAKISTERONE A (24-METHYL ECDYSONE)

B. Biosynthesis

Early work with labeled compounds demonstrated the in vivo conversion of injected cholesterol to ecdysone,[8] the high concentration of 7-dehydro-cholesterol in the prothoracic glands and the higher conversion of this sterol to ecdysone when compared to cholesterol.[148] In vivo metabolism of ecdysone to 20-hydroxyecdysone and of 22,25-dideoxyecdysone to the two ecdysteroids was also shown, and the intermediacy of 25-deoxyecdysone ruled out.[148] During the metabolism of cholesterol to ecdysone in blow fly larvae, the 7β hydrogen was lost[149] just as it was in the desaturation of cholesterol to 7-dehydrocholesterol in the same insect.[36] The 3α and 4β hydrogen atoms of cholesterol were lost during its conversion to 20-hydroxyecdysone in the locust which suggests a Δ^4-3-one intermediate in the metabolic sequence.[149a] 7-Dehydrocholesterol constituted from 25 to 60% of the total sterols in the prothoracic glands during pupation of the tobacco hornworm,[51] and was converted as readily as cholesterol to 20-hydroxyecdysone in locust larvae.[150] Cholesterol, 7-dehydrocholesterol, 3β,14α-dihydroxy-5β-cholest-7-en-6-one, and 22,25-dideoxyecdysone were all shown to be probable precursors of ecdysone in blow fly larvae. Inability of the larvae to metabolize 22- or 25-hydroxycholesterol suggested that some nuclear oxidations precede those in the side chain during ecdysone biosynthesis in some insects.[151]

In earlier stages of development, the 20-hydroxy group is missing in tobacco hornworm ecdysteroids. During the pupal-adult molt of this insect, 20-hydroxy and 20,26-dihydroxyecdysones are the principal ecdysteroids, whereas during embryogenesis, 26-hydroxyecdysone predominates.[152] An ecdysone 20-monooxygenase which uses cytochrome P-450 has been recently isolated from mitochondria of the tobacco hornworm fat body.[152a] This shows how biosynthetic pathways may be switched during different developmental stages of an insect. The isolation of 2-deoxyecdysone from ovaries and eggs of the silkworm showed that side chain hydroxylation may indeed take place before hydroxylation of the nucleus is complete and suggests that the 2-deoxy compound is the immediate precursor of ecdysone in vivo.[147]

The recent isolation of labeled 3β-hydroxy-5α-cholestan-6-one from silkworm prothoracic glands incubated with ^{14}C-cholesterol in vitro and the subsequent conversion

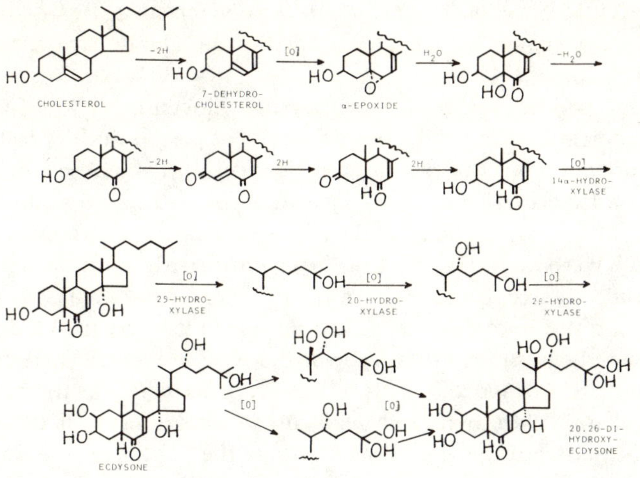

FIGURE 2. Possible biosynthetic pathways from cholesterol to ecdysteroids in insects.

of the saturated ketone to ecdysone by the same tissue reopened the question of the intermediacy of 7-dehydrocholesterol in ecdysteroid biosynthesis.[153] It is hard to reconcile both the $\Delta^{5,7}$-sterol[150] and the saturated ketone as common intermediates in the biosynthetic pathway. Other work with potential intermediates suggested the possible intermediacy of a 5β-hydroxy-Δ^7-6-one,[154] and a restudy of ecdysone biosynthesis with labeled (^{14}C-11,^{14}C-12) 3β-hydroxy-5α-cholest-7-en-6-one showed it to be incorporated into the hormone to much lesser degree (0.003%) than cholesterol (0.01-0.02%).[155]

Most of the steps in the biosynthesis appear to be specific mixed function oxidase catalyzed hydroxylations (C_2,C_{14},C_{20},C_{22},C_{25},C_{26}). The introduction of the 6-ketone may go through a 5α,6α-epoxide. Possible biosynthetic pathways, based on all information available at present, are shown in Figure 2.

C. Sites of Ecdysone Biosynthesis

The site of ecdysone biosynthesis was initially deduced from many surgical experiments with prothoracic glands and ecdysone assays on ligated animals. Larvae whose prothoracic glands had been removed failed to pupate; reimplantation of the tissue overcame this. The anterior portions of larvae that were ligated behind the prothoracic glands pupated, whereas the posterior portions (abdomens) maintained their larval cuticle and could even be severed from the anterior pupal forms for subsequent bioassays of ecdysteroid activity.

More recently, conflicting results were observed with isolated prothoracic glands. Although cholesterol was metabolized to ecdysone by prothoracic glands from larvae of the yellow mealworm[156] and 22,25-dideoxyecdysone was converted to ecdysone by prothoracic glands of tobacco hornworm larvae,[51] the absence of ecdysone biosynthesis in isolated prothoracic glands was reported in two other instances. Cholesterol was converted to ecdysone and 20-hydroxyecdysone in intact blow fly larvae but not when incubated with the brain-ring gland complex, tissue that includes the prothoracic glands of these insects.[157] In the second case, neither cholesterol nor 7-dehydrocholesterol were substrates for in vitro biosynthesis of ecdysone by prothoracic glands. Although the incorporation of lipoprotein into the culture medium increased ecdysone biosynthesis 10- to 20-fold, binding of ^{3}H-cholesterol to lipoprotein prior to its addition still did not convert it to ecdysone.[139] In addition, although 3β,14β-dihydroxy-5β-cholest-7-en-6-one was metabolized to ecdysone by prothoracic glands in vitro, the ketol, 3β-hydroxy-5β-cholest-7-en-6-one, was converted to 14-deoxyecdysone and other 14-deoxyecdysteroids, which indicated that the glands lack the enzyme systems for 14α-hydroxylation.[139]

The role of the prothoracic gland in ecdysone biosynthesis was first challenged in 1971. Ligation of armyworm larvae before a critical period in their last stage produced animals that had pupated anterior to the ligation and remained in the larval stage behind it. ^{3}H-Cholesterol was injected into these ligated larval abdomens and 6 days later unlabeled carriers were added and the tissues extracted. ^{3}H-Ecdysone and ^{3}H-20-hydroxyecdysone were identified by thin-layer chromatography on several solvents.[158]

A similar result was reported the following year. Abdomens, surgically removed from silkworms on the sixth day of the last larval stage, were injected with ^{14}C-cholesterol. After 24 hr, the tissues were homogenized with unlabeled carriers and crystalline ^{14}C-ecdysone and ^{14}C-20-hydroxy-ecdysone were isolated from them. Injection of labeled cholesterol into abdomens removed on the second day of the last larval stage did not yield labeled ecdysteroids. On this day, the prothoracic glands do not show histological activity in these insects, so it appeared that the glands are somehow involved in the biosynthetic process. The authors speculated that ecdysone is present in some bound form and that the prothoracic glands secrete a fluid at a certain time (day 5?) which catalyzes a step in the biosynthesis of ecdysone from cholesterol.[159] In other studies, the conversion of 3β,14α-dihydroxy-5β-cholest-7-en-6-one to 20-hydroxy-ecdysone occurred in isolated abdomens of blow fly larvae[151] and 22,25-deoxyecdysone is metabolized to 20-hydroxyecdysone and 20,26-dihydroxyecdysone when incubated with tobacco hornworm fat body or Malpighian tubules (excretory elements in insects).[51] During the last larval stage of the cabbageworm, however, no noticeable synthesis of ecdysone occurred in isolated abdomens. Ligation behind the head early in this stage kept the hemolymph ecdysone levels low and ligation behind the thorax later in the stage cut off the normal increase in ecdysone concentration that occurs in the hemolymph as the larvae mature.[160]

Conversion of cholesterol to ecdysone in several other tissues has been reported. Abdominal oenocytes removed from the last larval stage of the yellow mealworm metabolized ^{14}C-cholesterol mainly to 20-hydroxyecdysone, while the prothoracic glands from the same insect converted cholesterol only to ecdysone.[156] Oenocytes are cells of ectodermal origin found between the cuticle and basement membrane and are also associated with the fat body of insects. Maturing oocytes in silkworm pupae contain ecdysone; the concentration of the hormone in the eggs first increases during oocyte morphogenesis and then decreases at the end of the process.[161] A temperature sensitive mutant of *D. melanogaster,* which can reproduce normally at 20°C, becomes sterile at 29°C, at which temperature the ecdysone concentration in females is only 13% of that of the wild-type. When mutant ovaries are transplanted to wild-type females, they continue to develop at 20° but not at 29°C. The results suggest that ecdysone needed for female fertility is synthesized autonomously by ovarian tissues.[162] In another example, ovarian follicular cells of adult female locuts synthesized ecdysone during the terminal stages of oocyte maturation and transferred the hormone to the eggs where it was metabolized to more polar compounds. No ecdysteroids were found in ovariectomized females or adult males. Ovarian synthesis of ecdysone occurred even after removal of the prothoracic glands, and very little of the hormone was transferred to the blood or other tissues of the insect.[163] Ovarian increase in ecdysteroid concentration was prevented by removal of brain neurosecretory cells or corpora cardiaca from locusts, suggesting that ecdysone synthesis by ovarian tissue is stimulated by a neurohormone produced in the brain and secreted into the hemolymph by the corpora cardiaca.[164] In mosquito females, a brain hormone is implicated in the ovarian synthesis of ecdysone after a blood meal.[164a] In the final example, a large increase in ecdysone occurs after 6 to 10 days in isolated abdomens of yellow mealworm pupae and they undergo an adult molt. The authors suggest that prothoracic glands are required for ecdysone biosynthesis to stimulate larval-larval and larval-pupal molts, but that the pupal-adult metamorphosis is controlled by hormone synthesized in the abdomen, perhaps by oenocytes.[165]

In summary, both the sequence of reactions and the sites of ecdysteroid biosynthesis from cholesterol are still unclear. In spite of conflicting evidence, however, it appears that during larval stages, ecdysone synthesis is controlled by prothoracic glands. There may be several different biosynthetic pathways which respond to different regulators during the stages of the insects' maturation and reproduction processes.

D. Mechanism of Action

The modern concepts of steroid hormone-genome interaction originated in hypotheses first developed by Karlson and co-workers dealing with mechanisms of information transfer by ecdysone and supported by the correlation of "puffing" of the giant chromosomes in the salivary glands of certain insects with ecdysone titre. This was the first statement of the view now generally accepted that steroid hormones induce gene activities.[9,166]

The hypothesis that ecdysone interacts directly with DNA in insects to produce m-RNA and thereby induce protein synthesis was tested in several ways. The pupation of blow fly larvae, controlled by ecdysone, was delayed by injection of translation and transcription inhibitors when they were administered 20 hr, but not 8 or 69 hr before normal pupation. Ecdysone apparently induces the enzymes needed for pupation 20 hr before the event; by 8 hr before pupation they already exist and are not influenced by the inhibitors and when injected 69 hr before pupation, the inhibitors are metabolized before ecdysone becomes active.[166]

Ecdysone increased the turnover of RNA in epidermal tissue and enhanced the incorporation of ^{32}P-phosphate into ribosomal and messenger RNA. The m-RNA biosynthesized by ecdysone stimulation made more protein in vitro when incubated with insect or rat liver microsomes than the m-RNA from insects not treated with the hormone.[167] The nuclei from epidermal cells of blow fly larvae incorporated ^{14}C-uracil into RNA 2½ times more rapidly than controls when ecydsone was added to the in vitro incubation mixtures.[168] A portion of the RNA which is formed coded for DOPA-decarboxylase, an enzyme required for sclerotization of the newly formed cuticle.[9] Ecdysone, and to a greater extent, 20-hydroxy-ecdysone induces RNA synthesis in blow fly larval fat body cells and in the nuclei isolated from them. Most of the RNA synthesized is ribosomal RNA but some new species of nonribosomal RNA are also made under the influence of 20-hydroxy-ecdysone.[169]

The conversion of ecdysone to 20-hydroxyecdysone may be the initial target tissue response to ecdysone. Blow fly larval fat body responded only to 20-hydroxyecdysone and not to ecdysone for the initiation of RNA synthesis. This led Scheller and Karlson[169] to hypothesize that ecdysone is a prohormone and that 20-hydroxyecdysone is the real hormone for turning on protein synthesis in target tissues. The latter was the only ecdysteroid present in midge fly larvae (450 ng/g) just before pupation and its high concentration correlated with puffing at a particular site in the salivary chromosomes.[170] The hydroxylation of ecdysone to 20-hydroxyecdysone by preparations from Malpighian tubules and fat body of the desert locust was shown to require oxygen, cytochrome P450 and a mixed function oxidoreductase, and in this way, resembles the hydroxylation of steroids in mammalian systems.[171]

In summary, ecdysone acts as a typical steroid hormone. In response to an external stimulus, it is elicited by one tissue, travels in the blood to another where, after 20-hydroxylation, it is transported to the nucleus and acts directly on the genome. c-

AMP is not an intermediary in the process.[172] The RNA and subsequent proteins that result from this interaction control the physiological and morphological changes that take place in the insect.

A nonhormonal role for ecdysone was recently discovered in mosquitoes. Biting behavior by these insects is inhibited by ovarian development and by injected or ingested ecdysone. Ovariectomized fertilized mosquitoes still bite, but if ovaries are implanted, biting is inhibited.[173]

E. Biological Activity

Molting hormone activity of ecdysteroids is measured by injection of known quantities of these compounds into ligated abdomens whose anterior portion has pupated. The amount required to form a pupal epidermis in 50% of the injected larval abdomens is called "1 unit". By using the blow fly (larval wt. 36 mg), 1 unit of ecdysone was shown to be 0.01 μg of this hormone.[9] The smaller house fly larvae (16 mg) required only 0.005 μg ecdysone for the same response,[174] whereas the larger flesh fly larvae (55 mg) needed 0.035 μg of ecdysone for half of the ligated abdomens to form pupal cuticle.[175]

When 2β,3β,14α-trihydroxy-5β-cholest-7-en-6-one, which had 1/6 of the molting hormone activity of ecdysone by the house fly assay, was modified by preparation of the 2-acetate, 2,3-diacetate, saturation of the Δ^7-bond, elimination of the 14α-hydroxyl or the C_{27} carbon atom or by addition of a methyl or ethyl group at C_{24} in the side chain, the resulting compounds no longer possessed molting activity.[176] In addition, the conversion of the 5β(A/B rings *cis*) configuration to a 5α(A/B rings *trans*) eliminated all activity by the house fly assay.[176] Inversion of the configuration of the hydroxyl at C_{22} in ecdysone from 22R to 22S rendered 22-epiecdysone inactive by the house fly assay but allowed it to be still 1/8 to 1/4 as active as ecdysone in the cynthia moth caterpillar.[177] Taken all together, the evidence suggests that the 5β-Δ^7-6-ketone group is mandatory and that oxygens at C_3, C_{14} and C_{22} contribute most to the molting hormone activity of ecdysteroids. Oxygen atoms at C_2 and C_{25} are not as important, and an additional one at C_{26} reduces the activity of the hormone.

Ecdysteroids and analogs have also been tested as inhibitors of normal growth and development of insects. 3β-Hydroxy-5α-cholestan-6-one and the 2β-hydroxy (5α or 5β)-derivatives of this compound were the most active in preventing post-ecdysial hardening and sclerotization of the cuticle in the bug *Pyrrhocoris apterus* L. when 10 to 50 μg of ecdysone analogs were implanted in larval body cavities. They were considered to be ecdysone antagonists, and all of the active compounds tested in this study had 3β-hydroxy and 6-keto groups; the 5α or 5β-configuration was not important.[178] The quantities implanted were much larger than the normal concentration of ecdysteroids in insects, and one of the most active compounds in this test (3β-hydroxy-5α-cholestan-6-one) was later found to occur naturally in silkworm prothoracic glands and be a possible precursor to ecdysone.[153] The inhibitory effects of a large number of compounds related to ecdysone were also tested at various concentrations in the diets of house flies and several other insects.[176] The true ecdysteroids were largely noninhibitory in these tests, either because they were not absorbed or because of rapid deactivation by the insects. However recent work with house fly larvae reared on an axenic casein diet showed that ingestion of 100 ppm 20-hydroxyecdysone adversely affected growth and development.[176a] The compounds which inhibited growth and development the most were 22,25-dideoxyecdysone (ketotriol), its 2 and 2,3-di-0-methyl ethers and its 2,3-di-0-tri-methyl-silyl derivative. These compounds inhibited house fly larval maturation by 85 to 95% at a level of 75 μg/g and 60% at a level of

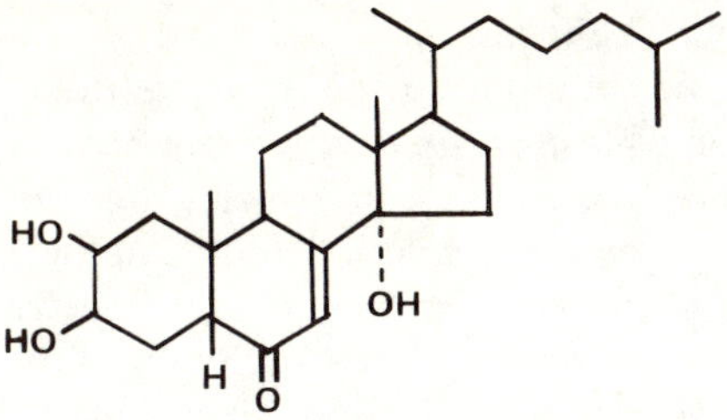

KETOTRIOL
(22,25-DIDEOXYECDYSONE)
(5α-CHOLEST-7-EN-2β,3β,14α-TRIOL-6-ONE)

15 μg/g in the diet. Larvae of other insects were similarly affected. The ketotriol caused 100% inhibition of maturation when 0.5% was added to the diet of the confused flour beetle, with 0.05% in the diet of the German cockroach and when 0.1 ppm was present in the water used for rearing yellow fever mosquitoes. Addition of much higher concentrations of the 5α-analogs of these active compounds to the various media did not inhibit growth and development of these four species of insects. Other inactive compounds included those lacking a 14α-hydroxyl group and those substituted with methyl or ethyl at C_{24} in the side chain.[176] It is noteworthy that the ecdysteroid analog most active as a growth inhibitor, the above ketotriol, is a compound that is probably an important intermediate in ecdysone biosynthesis by insects.[51,148,151] It apparently cannot be as efficiently inactivated as ecdysone or 20-hydroxyecdysone by the insects' intestinal tracts and is absorbed, possibly to inhibit ecdysone biosynthesis or to stimulate it at an inappropriate time.

F. Ecdysteroid Involvement in Reproduction

In addition to ecdysis, ecdysone and juvenile hormone are involved in reproductive processes. Numerous studies have shown how juvenile hormone is required for normal ovarian development;[179-181] yolk protein synthesis by fat body,[182-184] and oocyte maturation.[182] The role of ecdysteroids is not so clear. The ovarian synthesis of ecdysone in *D. melanogaster*[162] and a locust[163] and its transfer to the eggs of the latter insect correlate well with the isolation of 26-hydroxyecdysone from tobacco hornworm eggs[146] and of 2-deoxyecdysone from ovaries and eggs of the silkworm.[147] In locust eggs 95% of the ecdysteroids are in the conjugated form and do not get incorporated until the very end of egg development.[147a] In newly emerged mosquito adults, the development of oocytes is arrested after 3 days and remains suspended until blood is ingested. Injection of 20-hydroxyecdysone stimulated ovaries and initiated oogenesis in isolated mosquito abdomens, whereas two juvenile hormone analogs were inactive. Oral administration of 20-hydroxyecdysone to adult females (8 mg/g sucrose) also led to some oocyte production.[185] Cholesterol was used for ecdysone synthesis by the follicle cells of locust ovaries and a series of intermediates between the two steroids was detected by gas chromatography-mass spectroscopy.[186] Ecdysone passes into the terminal oocytes and is mostly conjugated in the embryo 2 to 3 days later. Both ecdysone and juvenile hormone promoted synthesis and secretion of egg yolk proteins in isolated abdomens of *D. melanogaster* but only juvenile hormone promoted their ovarian uptake and follicular development.[187] A feedback control of juvenile hormone synthesis by ecdysone has been suggested by recent work. When inactive female corpora allata were implanted into male cockroaches they became active and synthesized juvenile hormone. When ovaries were subsequently implanted into the males, juvenile hormone synthesis declined as oocytes completed maturation. Injection of ecdysone mimicked the effect of implanted ovaries.[187a]

In contrast to these findings, ecdysone was ineffective in stimulating ovarian development in tobacco hornworm larvae[179] and house fly adults.[180] It prevented the juvenile hormone stimulation of ovarian follicles in mosquito abdomens,[181] and rendered adult female stable flies completely sterile when the insects ingested a 0.1% solution of the hormone for 3 days.[188] Administration of ecdysone to the digestive tract of a bloodsucking bug inhibited oogenesis and oviposition in a dose dependant fashion. Doses greater than 4 ng/mg body weight reduced the size of the ovaries, but normal oviposition and oogenesis could be reestablished by a juvenile hormone analog.[189] It may be that ecdysone interaction with ovaries varies between insects and at different stages of an insect's development.[180] Its exact roles during reproduction are still not well understood.

The stimulation of spermatogenesis in the seminiferous tubules of mammals by testosterone has its counterpart in one study with insects. When intact testes from the cynthia moth were cultured in vitro with hemolymph plasma, no spermatogenesis occurred unless ecdysone was added to the medium. Other ecdysteroids and living, active prothoracic glands were also effective in inducing sperm to form.[190]

G. Catabolism and Excretion

Biological assay of extracts from the excreta of several insects showed that they contained ecdysteroids, and ecdysone was specifically identified in the fecal matter from locusts.[191] Excretion of ecdysteroid glycosides and sulfates by house flies has also been noted.[117] The metabolism of ecdysteroids to 3*β*-*α*-glucosides occurs in blow flies, whereas the principle products in the tobacco hornworm are the steroid sulfates.[117] Ecdysteroid fatty acid esters may also be involved in hormone deactivation reactions.[157] 20,26-Dihydroxyecdysone is less active than ecdysone or 20-hydroxyecdysone in one bioassay;[117] therefore, its presence in the tobacco hornworm[146] and a blow fly[192] may represent a deactivation product of the more potent hormones. The presence of 2-deoxyecdysone entirely as a conjugate in diapausing embryos indicated that ecdysteroid conjugates may be synthesized not only for excretion, but may also be storage forms of the hormones.[147]

The midgut of the tobacco hornworm contains other enzymes for ecdysone deactivation. Both 3-keto and 3*α*-hydroxyecdysones were identified after incubation of ecdysone with preparations from midgut tissue.[193] An enzyme isolated from blowfly pupae specifically oxidized ecdysteroids to 3-keto derivatives. Cholesterol oxidase and 3*α* and 3*β*-hydroxysteroid dehydrogenases were inactive in the assay.[194] From all these data, the catabolism of ecdysone can be represented as follows in various insects:

ECDYSONE

3-KETOECDYSONE

3-EPIECDYSONE

20-HYDROXYECDYSONE

20,26-DIHYDROXYECDYSONE

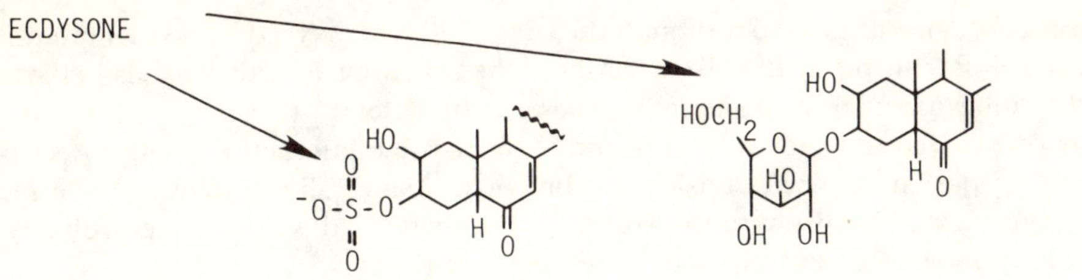

ECDYSONE

ECDYSONE 3-SULFATE

ECDYSONE 3-β-D-GLUCOSIDE

H. Phytoecdysteroids

The discovery of ecdysteroids in plants was probably one of the most unanticipated events in this field in recent times. The wood[195] and leaves[196] of two species of *Podocarpus* trees contained relatively large amounts of 20-hydroxyecdysone and 20-hydroxy-25-deoxyecdysone, respectively. Shortly thereafter, ecdysteroids were found in other plants and by now over 40 structurally distinct compounds have been discovered.[139,177] All are 5β-Δ^7-6-ketones, all but one have 2β,3β-hydroxyl groups and all but a few have a 14α-hydroxyl group. They differ in side chain hydroxylation and alkylation (methyl or ethyl) at C_{24}. Analysis of 1056 Japanese plants by dipping ligated rice stem borers into their methanol extracts showed ecdysteroid activity in 24 species of Pteridophytes and 30 species of Gymnosperms and Angiosperms (both mono- and dicots).[177] The compounds are therefore fairly widely distributed in the plant kingdom. The presence of ecdysteroids in plants does not inhibit insects from feeding on them[197] and incorporation of these compounds into the food of four species did not prevent the insects' growth or maturation.[176] The ecdysone and 20-hydroxyecdysone in bracken ferns appeared in the feces of the locusts eating these plants.[197] The reasons why some plants synthesize ecdysteroids and their function in plants are still unknown. The structures of a few representative plant ecdysteroids are:[177]

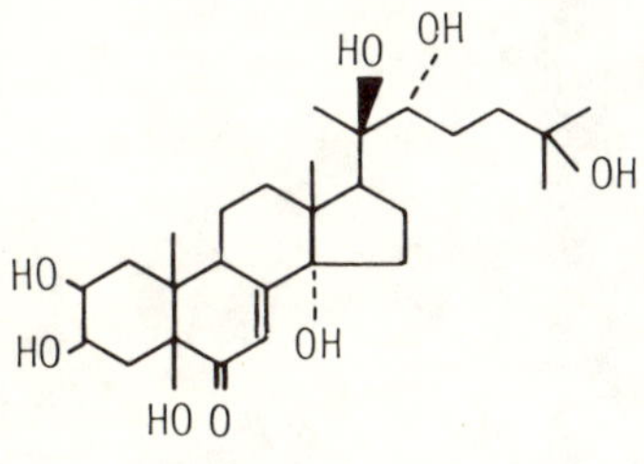

POLYPODINE-B

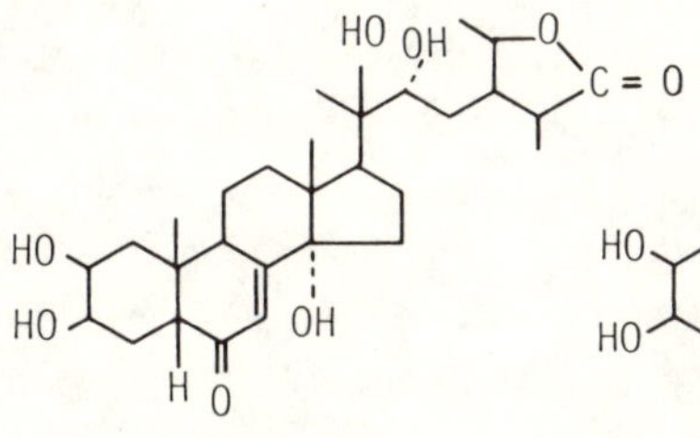

CYASTERONE

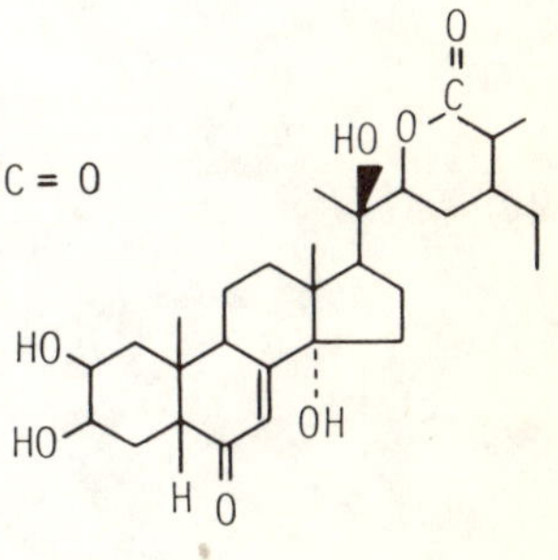

CAPITASTERONE

The biosynthesis of phytoecdysteroids may go through the same sequence of reactions from plant sterols that takes place in insects. Application of ^{14}C-cholesterol to the leaves of a *Podocarpus elatus* seedling led to radioactive 20-hydroxyecdysone whereas application of ^{14}C-cholest-4-en-3-one did not.[198] The 7β-hydrogen was lost from cholesterol during its conversion to 20-hydroxyecdysone in two plants just as it was during its conversion to ecdysone in an insect.[149]

I. Summary

The synthesis of ecdysteroids has been shown to take place in three different tissues of insects, the prothoracic glands, oenocytes and ovaries, as well as in over 40 different species of plants. Their concentrations change during various stages of maturation and reproduction in insects, and although the role of 20-hydroxyecdysone as a molting and metamorphosis hormone is well established, the functions of ecdysteroids in the ovary, oocyte, embryo, and during spermatogenesis are not clear.

The role of ecdysteroids in plants and their possible interactions with insect predators in the past have been considered, but no evidence shows deleterious effects of plant concentrations of phytoecdysteroids on insects. Ecdysteroids are probably used as molting hormones by all modern arthropods (insects, spiders, millipedes, crabs, lobsters, etc) and may go back to a common ancestor of these organisms which existed 500 million years ago.[199]

APPENDIX 1

INSECTS MENTIONED IN TEXT AND IN THE LITERATURE REFERENCES

Common Names	Scientific Names
A	
Ambrosia beetle	*Xyloborus ferrugineus*
American cockroach	*Periplaneta americana*
Angoumois grain moth	*Sitotroga cerealella*
Armyworm	*Mamestra brassicae*
B	
Bean weevil	*Acanthoscellides obtectus*
Black blow fly	*Phormia regina*
Black carpet beetle	*Attagenus picius*
Blood sucking bug	*Rhodius prolixus*
Blow flies	*Calliphora erythrocephala (= C. vicina)*
	Calliphora stygia
	Lucilia sericata
Boll weevil	*Anthonomus grandis*
C	
Cabbage butterfly	*Pieris brassicae*
Cabbage root fly	*Hylema brassicae*
Cecropia moth	*Hyalophora cecropia*
Chrysomelid beetles	*In genera: Chrysolina,*
	Chrysochloa
	Diochrysa
Cigarette beetle	*Lasioderma sericorne*
Clothes moth	*Tineola bisselliella*
Cockroaches	*Eurycotis floridana*
	Leucophaea maderae
	Nauphoeta cinerea
Colorado potato beetle	*Leptinotarsa decemlineata*
Confused flour beetle	*Tribolium confusum*
Corn borer	*Pyrausta nubilialis*
Corn earworm	*Heliothis zea*
Cotton leafworm	*Spodoptera littoralis (Boisduval)*
Cynthia moth	*Samia cynthia*
D	
Dipteran entomophagous parasite	*Pseudosarcophaga affinis*
Drugstore beetles	*Sitodrepa panicea*
	Stegobium paniceum

E

Endoparasitoid wasp	*Itoplectis conquisitor*

F

Fall armyworm	*Spodoptera frugiperda*
Firebrat	*Thermobia domestica*
Flesh flies	*Sarcophaga bullata*
	Sarcophaga peregrina
Fruit flies	*Drosophila funebris*
	Drosophila immigrans
	Drosophila melanogaster
	Drosophila pachea

G

German cockroach	*Blattella germanica*
Grasshoppers	*Melanoplus bivittatus*
	Poekilocerus bufonius (Klug)

H

Hide beetle	*Dermestes vulpinis (= D. maculatus)*
Honey bee	*Apis mellifera (= A. mellifica)*
House cricket	*Acheta domesticus (= Gryllus domesticus)*
House flies	*Musca domestica*
	Musca vicina

I

Ichneumenoid parasitic wasp	*Hyposoter exiguae*

K

Khapra beetle	*Trogoderma granarium*

L

Locusts	*Locusta migratoria*
	Schistocerca gregaria (Forskal)

M

Mediterranean flour moth	*Anagasta kuhniella Z. (= Ephestia k.Z.)*
Mexican bean beetle	*Epilachna varivestis*
Midge fly	*Chironomus thummi*
Milkweed bug	*Oncopeltus fasciatus (Dallas)*
Monarch butterfly	*Danaus plexippus*
Mopani moth	*Gonimbrasia belina*
Mormon cricket	*Anabrus simplex*
Mosquitoes	*Aedes aegypti*
	Anopheles quadrimaculatus
	Culex pipiens quinquefasciatus

Moth	*Crambus trisectus (Walker)*
O	
Oriental hornet	*Vespa orientalis*
Oriental house fly	*Musca domestica vicina*
P	
Pales (pine) beetle	*Hylobius pales*
Pyrrhocorid bug	*Pyrrhocoris apterus*
R	
Rice moth	*Corcyra cephalonica*
Rice stem borer	*Chilo simplex*
S	
Sawtoothed grain beetle	*Silvanus (Oryzaephilus) surinamensis*
Screwworm	*Cochliomyia hominivorax (Coquerel)*
Silkworms	*Bombyx mori*
Silverfish	*Ctenolepisma* sp.
	Lepisma saccharina
Smaller brown plant hopper	*Laodelphax striatellus*
Southern cowpea weevil	*Callosobruchus chinensis*
Southwestern corn borer	*Diatraea grandiosella*
Spider beetle	*Ptinus tectus*
Stable fly	*Stomoxys calcitrans*
T	
Termite	*Macrotermes goliath*
Tea tortrix	*Homona coffearia*
Tobacco hornworm	*Manduca sexta*
V	
Virginia pine sawfly	*Neodiprion pratti*
W	
Water beetles	*Acilius sulcatus*
	Cybister sp.
	Dysticsus marginalis
Wax moth	*Galleria melonella*
Weevil	*Anthomonus pernyi*
Wood boring beetle	*Hylotrupes bajulus*
Y	
Yellow mealworm	*Tenebrio molitor*

APPENDIX 2

STEROL NOMENCLATURE

Sterols are referred to in the text, tables and references by trivial and systematic names. The systematic nomenclature used here is based on the following stem names:

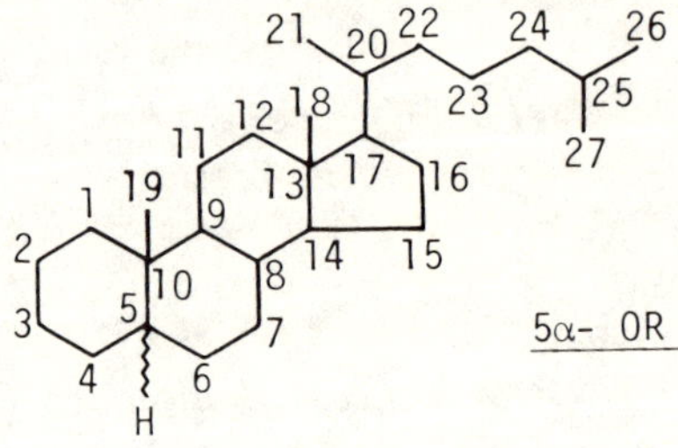

5α- OR 5β-CHOLESTANE

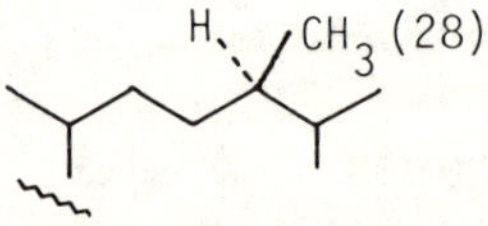

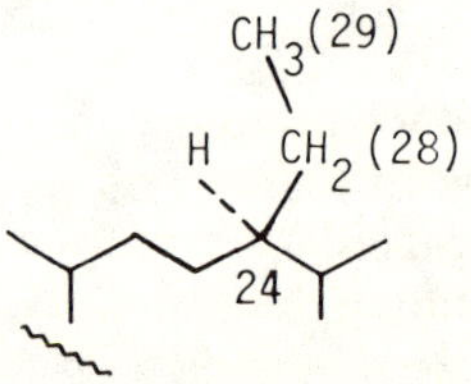

24 α CAMPESTANE STIGMASTANE

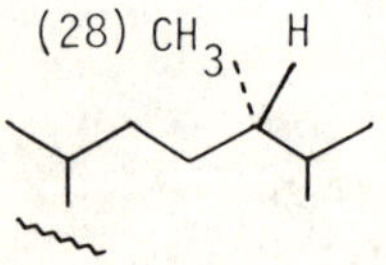

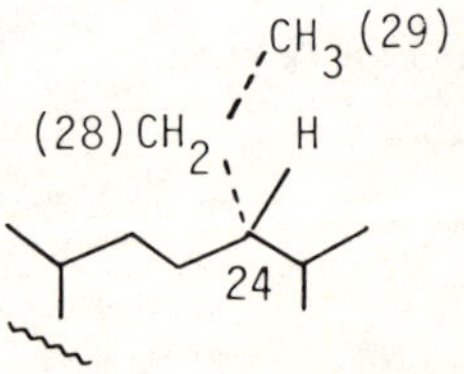

24 β ERGOSTANE PORIFERASTANE

GLOSSARY OF STEROL NAMES

Trivial Names	Systematic Names
Brassicasterol	Ergosta-5,22E-dien-3β-ol
Calciferol	9,10-*Seco*-Cholesta-5,7,10(19)-trien-3β-ol
Campestanol	5α-Campestan-3β-ol
7-Campestenol	5α-Campest-7-en-3β-ol
Campesterol	Campest-5-en-3β-ol
Cholestanol	5α-Cholestan-3β-ol
Cholestanone	5α-Cholestan-3-one
Cholestenone	Cholest-4-en-3-one
Cholesterol	Cholest-5-en-3β-ol
Clerosterol	Poriferasta-5,25-dien-3β-ol
Clionasterol	Poriferast-5-en-3β-ol
Cycloartenol	9,19-*cyclo*-Lanost-24-en-3β-ol
Coprostanol	5β-Cholestan-3β-ol
7-Coprostenol	5β-Cholest-7-en-3β-ol
Cybisterol	Pregna-4,6-dien-11β-ol-3,20-dione
7-Dehydrocholesterol	Cholesta-5,7-dien-3β-ol
22-Dehydrocholesterol	Cholesta-5,22E-dien-3β-ol
22-Dehydrodesmosterol	Cholesta-5,22E,24-trien-3β-ol
Dehydroepiandrosterone	Androst-5-en-3β-ol-17-one
7-Dehydrositosterol	Stigmasta-5,7-dien-3β-ol
Desmosterol	Cholesta-5,24-dien-3β-ol
20,25-Diazacholesterol	20,25-Diazacholest-5-en-3β-ol
22,25-Diazacholesterol	22,25-Diazacholest-5-en-3β-ol
Dihydrobrassicasterol	Ergost-5-en-3β-ol
4,4′-Dimethyl-8-cholestenol	4,4′-Dimethyl-5α-cholest-8(9)-en-3β-ol
Ecdysone	(22R)-2β,3β,14,22,25-Pentahydroxy-5β-cholest-7-en-6-one
22-Epiecdysone	(22S)-2β,3β,14,22,25-Pentahydroxy-5β-cholest-7-en-6-one
Ergocalciferol	9,10-*Seco*-Ergosta-5,7,10(19),22E-tetraene-3β-ol
5,7-Ergostadienol	Ergosta-5,7-dien-3β-ol
7,22-Ergostadienol	5α-Ergosta-7,22E-dien-3β-ol
Ergostanol	5α-Ergostan-3β-ol
7-Ergostenol	5α-Ergost-7-en-3β-ol
Ergosterol	Ergosta-5,7,22E-trien-3β-ol
Fucosterol	Stigmasta-5,24(28)E-dien-3β-ol
3α-Hydroxyecdysone	(22R)-2β,3α,14,22,25-Pentahydroxy-5β-cholest-7-en-6-one
Isofucosterol	Stigmasta-5,24(28)Z-dien-3β-ol
3-Ketoecdysone	(22R)-2β,14,22,25-Tetrahydroxy-5β-cholest-7-en-3,6-dione
Lanosterol	5α-Lanosta-8(9),24-dien-3β-ol
Lathosterol	5α-Cholest-7-en-3β-ol
Lophenol	4α-Methyl-5α-cholest-7-en-3β-ol
Lumisterol	10α-Cholesta-5,7-dien-3β-ol
24-Methylenecholesterol	Ergosta-5,24(28)-dien-3β-ol
Makisterone A	(22R)-2β,3β,14,20,22,25-Hexa-hydroxy-5β-campest-7-en-6-one

Progesterone	Pregn-4-en-3,20-dione
Pregnenolone	Pregn-5-en-3β-ol-20-one
Schottenol	5α-Stigmast-7-en-3β-ol
Sitosterol	Stigmast-5-en-3β-ol
Stigmastanol	5α-Stigmastan-3β-ol
22-Stigmastenol	5α-Stigmast-22E-en-3β-ol
Stigmasterol	Stigmasta-5,22E-dien-3β-ol
Testosterone	Androst-4-en-3-on-17β-ol
Zymosterol	5α-Cholesta-8(9),24-dien-3β-ol

GLOSSARY OF OTHER NAMES

General Name	Example	Systematic Name
Androgen	Dihydrotestosterone	5β-Androstan-3-on-17β-ol
Bile acid	Cholic acid	3α,7α,12α-trihydroxy-5β-cholan-24-oic acid
Bile alcohol	Scymnol	3α,7α,12α,24ξ,26,27-Hexahydroxy-5β-cholestane
Bufadienolide	Bufalin	3β,14-Dihydroxy-5β,14β-bufa-20,22-dienolide
Cardenolide	Digitoxigenin	3β,14-Dihydroxy-5β,14β-card-20(22)-en-olide
Cardiac glycoside	Digitoxin	Trisaccharide 3-β-D-glycoside of digi-toxigenin
Corticoid	Cortisone	Pregn-4-en-17,21-diol-3,11,20-trione
Estrogen	Estradiol	Estra-1,3,5(10)-trien-3,17β-diol
Juvagen	Juvenile hormone	Methyl 3,11-dimethyl-7-ethyl-10,11-epoxy-trideca-2E,6E-dienoate
Progestagen	Progesterone	Pregn-4-en-3,20-dione
Sapogenin	Diosgenin	(25R)-Spirost-5-en-3β-ol
Steroid alkaloid	Tomatidine	(22R,25R)-5α-tomatanine-3β-ol
Triparanol (MER-29)	—	1-[p-(2-diethylamino-ethoxy) phenyl]-1-(p-tolyl)-2-(p-chlorophenyl)-ethanol

REFERENCES

1. **Hobson, R. P.,** On a fat soluble growth factor required by blowfly larvae. II. Indentity of the growth factor with cholesterol, *Biochem. J.*, 29, 2023, 1935.
2. **Van't Hoog, E. G.,** Aseptic culture of insects in vitamin research, *Z. Vitam. Forsch.*, 5, 118, 1936.
3. **Lipke, H. and Frankel, G.,** Insect nutrition, *Ann. Rev. Entomol.*, 1, 17, 1956.
4. **Clayton, R. B.,** The utilization of sterols by insects, *J. Lipid Res.*, 5, 3, 1964.
5. **Clark, A. J. and Bloch, K.,** The absence of sterol synthesis in insects, *J. Biol. Chem.*, 234, 2578, 1959.
6. **Clark, A. J. and Bloch, K.,** Function of sterols in *Dermestes vulpinus*, *J. Biol. Chem.*, 234, 2583, 1959.
7. **Clark, A. J. and Bloch, K.,** Conversion of ergosterol to 22-dehydro-cholesterol in *Blattella germanica*, *J. Biol. Chem.*, 234, 2589, 1959.
8. **Karlson, P. and Hoffmeister, H.,** Biogenesis of ecdysone, I. Conversion of cholesterol to ecdysone, *Z. Physiol. Chem.*, 331, 298, 1963.
9. **Karlson, P.,** Ecdysone, the molting hormone of insects, *Die Naturwiss.*, 21b, 445, 1966.
10. **Clayton, R. B., Edwards, A. M., and Bloch, K.,** Biosynthesis of cholesterol in an insect, silverfish (*Ctenolepisma* sp.), *Nature*, 193, 1125, 1962.
11. **Noda, H., Wada, K., and Saito, T.,** Sterols in *Laodelphax striatellus* with special reference to the intracellular yeast-like symbiotes as a sterol source, *J. Insect Physiol.*, 25, 443, 1979.
12. **Kaplanis, J. N., Robbins, W. E., Vroman, H. E., and Bryce, B. M.,** The absence of cholesterol biosynthesis in a primitive insect, the firebrat *Thermobia domestica* (Packard), *Steroids*, 2, 547, 1963.
13. **Zandee, D. I.,** Absence of sterol synthesis in some arthropods, *Nature*, 202, 1335, 1964.
14. **Teshima, S. I. and Kanazawa, A.,** Biosynthesis of sterols in the lobster, *Panulirus japonica*, the prawn, *Penaeus japonicus* and the crab, *Portunus trituberculatus*, *Comp. Biochem. Physiol.*, 38B, 597, 1971.
15. **Levinson, Z. H. and Bergmann, E. D.,** Steroid utilization and fatty acid synthesis by larva of the housefly, *Musca vicina Macq.*, *Biochem. J.*, 65, 254, 1957.
16. **Dwivedy, A. K.,** Dietary cholesterol requirements of the housefly, *Musca domestica*, larvae, *J. Insect Physiol.*, 21, 1685, 1975.
17. **Dambrae-Raes, H.,** The effect of dietary cholesterol on the development of *Hylema brassicae*, *J. Insect Physiol.*, 22, 287, 1976.
18. **Earle, N. W., Walker, A. B., and Burks, M. L.,** Storage and excretion of steroids in the adult boll weevil, *Comp. Biochem. Physiol.*, 16, 277, 1965.
19. **Frankel, G. and Blewett, M.,** The sterol requirements of several insects, *Biochem. J.*, 37, 692, 1943.
20. **Noland, J. L.,** I. Utilization of cholesterol derivatives by the German cockroach, *Blattella germanica*, *Arch. Biochem. Biophys.*, 48, 370, 1954. II. Inhibition of cholesterol utilization by structural analogs, 52, 323, 1954.
21. **Dadd, R. H.,** The nutritional requirements of locusts. II. Utilization of sterols, *J. Insect Physiol.*, 5, 161, 1960.
22. **Gilmour, D.,** *The Biochemistry of Insects*, Academic Press, New York, 1961, 32.
23. **Clayton, R. B. and Edwards, A. M.,** The essential cholesterol requirement of the roach *Eurycotis floridana*, *Biochem. Biophys. Res. Comm.*, 6, 281, 1961.
24. **Morisaki, M., Ohtaka, H., Kubayashi, M., Ikekawa, N., Horie, Y., and Nakasone, S.,** Fucosterol-24,28-epoxide as a probable intermediate in the conversion of β-sitosterol to cholesterol in the silkworm, *J. Chem. Soc., Chem. Comm.*, 1275, 1972.
25. **Gingrich, R. E.,** Nutritional studies on screw worm larvae with chemically defined media, *Ann. Ent. Soc. Am.*, 57, 351, 1964.
26. **Royes, V. W. and Robertson, F. W.,** The nutritional requirements and growth relations of different species of Drosophila, *J. Exptl. Zool.*, 156, 105, 1964.
27. **Vroman, H. E., Kaplanis, J. N., and Robbins, W. E.,** Cholesterol turnover in the American cockroach, *Periplaneta americana*, *J. Lipid Res.*, 5, 418, 1964.
28. **Kaplanis, J. N., Robbins, W. E., Monroe, R. E., Shortino, T. J., and Thompson, M. J.,** The utilization and fate of β-sitosterol in the larvae of the housefly, *Musca domestica*, *J. Insect Physiol.*, 11, 251, 1965.

28a. **Herbert, E. W., Jr., Svoboda, J. A., Thompson, M. J., and Shimanuki, H.,** Sterol utilization in honey bees fed a synthetic diet: Effects on brood rearing, *J. Insect Physiol.*, 26, 287, 1980.

28b. **Herbert, E. W., Jr., Svoboda, J. A., Thompson, M. J., and Shimanuki, H.,** Sterol utilization in honey bees fed a synthetic diet: Analysis of prepupal sterols, *J. Insect Physiol.*, 26, 291, 1980.

29. **Svoboda, J. A. and Robbins, W. E.,** Conversion of beta-sitosterol to cholesterol blocked in an insect by hypercholesterolemic agents, *Science*, 156, 1637, 1967.
30. **Agarwal, H. C.,** Sterol requirements of the beetle *Trogoderma*, *J. Insect Physiol.*, 16, 2023, 1970.

31. **Goodfellow, R. D., Barnes, F. J., and Graham, W. T., Jr.,** Dietary sterol effects on mevalonate kinase activity in axenic and non-axenic *Sarcophaga bullata* (Diptera), *J. Insect Physiol.*, 17, 1625, 1971.
32. **Chippendale, G. M.,** Lipid requirements of the angoumois grain moth, *Sitotroga cerealella, J. Insect Physiol.*, 17, 2169, 1971.
33. **Chippendale, G. M. and Reddy, G. P. V.,** Polyunsaturated fatty acid and sterol requirements of the southwestern corn borer, *Diatraea grandiosella, J. Insect Physiol.*, 18, 305, 1972.
34. **Yazgan, S.,** A chemically defined synthetic diet and larval nutritional requirements of the endoparasitoid, *Ictoplectis conquisitor, J. Insect Physiol.*, 18, 2123, 1972.
35. **Richmond, J. A. and Thomas, H. A.,** *Hylobius pales*, effect of dietary sterols on development and on sterol content of somatic tissue, *Ann. Ent. Soc. Am.*, 68, 329, 1975.
36. **Johnson, P., Cook, I. F., Rees, H. H., and Goodwin, T. W.,** Mode of formation of cholesta-5,7-dien-3β-ol from cholest-5-en-3β-ol by larvae of *Calliphora erythrocephala, Biochem. J.*, 152, 303, 1975.
37. **Cooke, J. and Sang, J. H.,** Utilization of sterols by larvae of *Drosophila melanogaster, J. Insect Physiol.*, 16, 801, 1970.
38. **Gordan, H. T.,** Minimal nutritional requirements of the German cockroach, *Blattella germanica* L., *N.Y. Acad. Sci.*, 77, 290, 1959.
39. **Beck, S. D. and Kapadia, G. G.,** Sterols in confused flour beetle *(Tribolium confusum), Science*, 126, 258, 1957.
40. **Dutky, R. C., Robbins, W. E., Shortino, T. J., Kaplanis, J. N., and Vroman, H. E.,** The conversion of cholestanone to cholestanol by the housefly, *Musca domestica* L., *J. Insect Physiol.*, 13, 1501, 1967.
41. **Morisaki, M., Ohtaka, H., Awata, N., Ikekawa, N., Horie, Y., and Nakasone, S.,** Nutritional effect of possible intermediates of phytosterol dealkylation in the silkworm, *Bombyx mori, Steroids*, 24, 165, 1974.

41a. **Nicotra, F., Ronchetti, F., Russo, G., and Toma, L.,** Role of 24- and 28-hydroxylated intermediates in the metabolism of β-sitosterol in the insect *Tenebrio molitor, Biochem. J.*, 183, 495, 1979.

42. **Katz, M., Budowski, P., and Bondi, A.,** The effect of phytosterols on the growth and sterol composition of *Dermestes maculatus, J. Insect Physiol.*, 17, 1295, 1971.
43. **Levinson, Z. H.,** The function of dietary sterols in phytophagous insects, *J. Insect Physiol.*, 8, 191, 1962.

43a. **Thompson, S. N.,** *Brachymeria lasus* and *Pachycrepoideus vindemiae:* Sterol requirements during larval growth of two hymenopterous insect parasites reared *in vitro* on chemically defined media, *Exptl. Parasitol.*, 51, 220, 1981.

43b. **Ritter, K. S. and Nes, W. R.,** The effects of cholesterol on the development of *Heliothis zea, J. Insect Physiol.*, 27, 175, 1981.

43c. **Ritter, K. S. and Nes, W. R.,** The effects of the structure of sterols on the development of *Heliothis zea, J. Insect Physiol.*, 27, 419, 1981.

44. **Ito, T.,** Sterol requirement of the silkworm, *Bombyx mori, Nature*, 191, 882, 1961.
45. **Ito, T. and Horie, Y.,** Utilization of sterols and related compounds by the silkworm, *Bombyx mori* L., *Ann. Zool. Jpn.*, 39, 1, 1966.
46. **Dupnik, D. T. and Kamm, J. A.,** Development of an artificial diet for *Crambus trisectus, J. Econ. Entomol.*, 63, 1578, 1970.
47. **Chu, H-M., Norris, D. M., and Kok, L. T.,** Pupation requirement for the beetle *Xyloborus ferrugineus:* sterols other than cholesterol, *J. Insect Physiol.*, 16, 1379, 1970.

47a. **Norris, D. M. and Moore, C. L.,** Lack of a Δ^7-sterol markedly shortens the periods of locomotor vigor, reproduction and longevity of adult female *Xyloborus ferrugineus (Coleoptera, Scolytidae), Expt. Geront.*, 15, 359, 1980.

48. **Heed, W. B. and Kircher, H. W.,** Unique sterol in the ecology and nutrition of *Drosophila pachea, Science*, 149, 758, 1965.
49. **Sivapalan, P. and Gnanapragasam, N. C.,** The influence of linoleic acid and linolenic acid on adult moth emergence of *Homona coffearia* from meridic diets in vitro, *J. Insect Physiol.*, 25, 393, 1979.
50. **Earle, N. W., Lambremont, E. N., Burks, M. L., Slatten, B. H., and Bennett, A. F.,** Conversion of β-sitosterol to cholesterol in the boll weevil and inhibition of larval development by two aza sterols, *J. Econ. Entomol.*, 60, 291, 1967.
51. **Thompson, M. J., Kaplanis, J. N., Robbins, W. E., and Svoboda, J. A.,** Metabolism of steroids in insects, *Adv. Lipid Res.*, 11, 219, 1973.
52. **Svoboda, J. A. and Robbins, W. E.,** Desmosterol as a common intermediate in the conversion of a number of C_{28} and C_{29} plant sterols to cholesterol by the tobacco hornworm, *Experientia*, 24, 1131, 1968.
53. **Nair, A. M. G. and Agarwal, H. C.,** Sterols and sterol esters in nutrition of the beetle *Trogoderma granariun* Everts, *Indian J. Exptl. Biol.*, 15, 576, 1977.

54. **Salama, H. S. and El-Sharaby, A. M.**, Gibberelic acid and β-sitosterol as sterilants of cotton leafworm, *Spodoptera littoralis* Boisduval (a moth), *Experientia*, 28, 413, 1972.
55. **Kircher, H. W. and Gray, M. A.**, Cholestanol-cholesterol utilization by axenic *Drosophila melanogaster, J. Insect Physiol.*, 24, 555, 1978.
56. **Kircher, H. W.**, unpublished work.
57. **Ikan, R., Markus, A., and Bergmann, E. D.**, Synthesis of campesterol ((24R)-24-methyl-3β-acetoxycholest-5-ene) and its 24S-epimer, *Steroids*, 16, 517, 1970.
58. **Svoboda, J. A. and Robbins, W. E.**, 24-Methylenecholesterol: isolation and identification as an intermediate in the conversion of campesterol to cholesterol in the tobacco hornworm, *Lipids*, 7, 156, 1972.
59. **Svoboda, J. A., Thompson, M. J., and Robbins, W. E.**, Desmosterol, an intermediate in the dealkylation of β-sitosterol in the tobacco hornworm, *Life Sci.*, 6, 395, 1967.
60. **Clayton, R. B. and Bloch, K.**, Sterol utilization in the hide beetle, *Dermestes vulpinis, J. Biol. Chem.*, 238, 586, 1963.
61. **Clayton, R. B.**, unpublished work cited in Reference 4.
62. **Awata, N., Morisaki, M., Fujimoto, Y., and Ikekawa, N.**, Inhibitory effects of steroidal allenes on the growth, development and steroid metabolism of the silkworm, *Bombyx mori, J. Insect Physiol.*, 22, 403, 1976.
63. **Fujimoto, Y., Morisaki, M., Ikekawa, N., Horie, Y., and Nakasone, S.**, Synthesis of 24,28-iminofucosterol and its inhibitory effects on growth and steroid metabolism in the silkworm, *Bombyx mori, Steroids*, 24, 367, 1974.
64. **Bergmann, E. D., Rabinowitz, M., and Levinson, Z. H.**, The synthesis and biological activity of some lower homologs of cholesterol, *J. Am. Chem. Soc.*, 81, 1239, 1959.
64a. **Thompson, M. J., Patterson, G. W., Dutky, S. R., Svoboda, J. A., and Kaplanis, J. N.**, Techniques for the isolation and identification of sterols in insects and in algae, *Lipids*, 15, 719, 1980.
65. **Kircher, H. W., Heed, W. B., Russell, J. S., and Grove, J.**, Senita cactus alkaloids: Their significance to Sonoran Desert *Drosophila* ecology, *J. Insect Physiol.*, 13, 1869, 1967.
66. **Kircher, H. W.**, The distribution of sterols, alkaloids, and fatty acids in senita cactus, *Lophocereus schottii* (Engelmann) Britton and Rose, over its range in Sonora, Mexico, *Phytochemistry*, 8, 1481, 1969.
67. **Campbell, C. E. and Kircher, H. W.**, Senita cactus: A plant with interrupted sterol biosynthetic pathways, *Phytochemistry*, 19, 2777, 1980.
68. **Louloudes, S. J., Thompson, M. J., Monroe, R. E., and Robbins, W. E.**, Conversion of cholestanol to Δ^7-cholestenol by the German cockroach, *Biochem. Biophys. Res. Comm.*, 8, 104, 1962.
69. **Monroe, R. E.**, Role of cholesterol in house fly reproduction, *Nature*, 184, 1513, 1959.
70. **Kaplanis, J. N., Robbins, W. E., and Tabor, L. A.**, The utilization and metabolism of 4-^{14}C-cholesterol by the adult house fly, *Ann. Ent. Soc. Am.*, 53, 260, 1960.
71. **Monroe, R. E., Polityka, C. S., and Lamb, N. J.**, Utilization of larval cholesterol-4-^{14}C for reproduction in house flies fed unlabeled cholesterol in the adult diet, *Ann. Ent. Soc. Am.*, 61, 292, 1968.
72. **Norris, D. M. and Chu, H-M.**, Maternal *Xyloborus ferrugineus* transmission of sterol or sterol-dependent metabolites necessary for progeny pupation, *J. Insect Physiol.*, 17, 1741, 1971.
73. **Thompson, A. C., Henson, R. D., Gueldner, R. C., and Hedin, P. A.**, Sterol galactosides and sterol esters of the cotton bud, *Lipids*, 5, 283, 1970.
74. Abu-Mustafa, Constituents of local plants. VIII. Sterol content of the fat unsaponifiable fraction of twenty plant species, *J. Chem. U.A.R.*, 9, 93, 1966; *Chem. Abst.*, 67, 18546a, 1967.
75. **Kircher, H. W. and Rosenstein, F. U.**, Purification of sitosterol, *Lipids*, 8, 97, 1973.
76. **Goodnight, K. C. and Kircher, H. W.**, Metabolism of lathosterol by *Drosophila pachea, Lipids*, 6, 166, 1971.
77. **Thompson, M. J., Louloudes, S. J., Robbins, W. E., Waters, J. A., Steele, J. A., and Mosettig, E.**, The identify of the major sterol from houseflies reared by the CSMA procedure, *J. Insect Physiol.*, 9, 615, 1963.
78. **Clayton, R. B., Hinkle, P. C., Smith, D. A., and Edwards, A. M.**, The intestinal absorption of cholesterol, its esters and some related sterols and analogs in the roach, *Eurycotis floridana, Comp. Biochem. Physiol.*, 11, 333, 1964.
79. **Lasser, N. L., Edwards, A. M., and Clayton, R. B.**, Distribution and dynamic state of sterols and steroids in the tissues of an insect, the roach *Eurycotis floridana, J. Lipid Res.*, 7, 403, 1966.
79a. **Svoboda, J. A., Nair, A. M. G., Agarwal, N., and Robbins, W. E.**, The sterols of the Kapra beetle, *Trogoderma granarium* Everts, *Experientia*, 35, 1454, 1979.
80. **Svoboda, J. A., Dutky, S. R., Robbins, W. E., and Kaplanis, J. N.**, Sterol composition and phytosterol utilization and metabolism in the milkweed bug, *Lipids*, 12, 318, 1977.
80a. **Svoboda, J. A., Herbert, E. W., Jr., Thompson, M. J., and Shimanuki, H.**, The fate of radiolabelled C_{28} and C_{29} phytosterols in the honey bee, *J. Insect Physiol.*, 27, 183, 1981.

80b. **Svoboda, J. A., Nair, A. M. G., Agarwal, N., and Robbins, W. E.,** Lack of conversion of C_{29}-phytosterols to cholesterol in the Kapra beetle *Trogoderma granarium* Everts, *Experientia,* 36, 1029, 1980.

81. **Budowski, P., Ishaaya, I., and Katz, M.,** Growth inhibition of *Dermestes maculatus* by phytosterols, *J. Nutr.,* 91, 201, 1967.

82. **Ito, T. and Nakasone, S.,** Nutrition of the silkworm, *Bombyx mori*-XV. Utilization of sterol in the presence of dietary fatty acids, *J. Insect Physiol.,* 13, 281, 1967.

83. **Casida, J. E., Beck, S. D., and Cole, M. J.,** Sterol metabolism in the American cockroach, *J. Biol. Chem.,* 224, 365, 1957.

84. **Ikan, R., Gottlieb, R., and Bergmann, E. D.,** Lipids of the queen of the oriental hornet, *Vespa orientalis, J. Insect Physiol.,* 15, 1249, 1969.

85. **Wang, C. M., and Patton, R. L.,** Lipids in the haemolymph of the cricket *Acheta domesticus, J. Insect Physiol.,* 15, 851, 1969.

86. **Cmelik, S. H. W.,** The neutral lipids from various organs of the termite *Macrotermes goliath, J. Insect Physiol.,* 15, 839, 1969.

87. **Kinsella, J. E.,** The lipids of *Lepisma saccharina* L. (silverfish), *Lipids,* 4, 299, 1969.

88. **Ichimasa, Y.,** Sterol accumlation in developing ovaries of the silkworm, *Bombyx mori, J. Insect Physiol.,* 22, 1071, 1976.

89. **Monroe, R. E., Hopkins, T. L., and Valder, S. A.,** Metabolism and utilization of cholesterol-4-^{14}C for growth and reproduction of asceptically reared houseflies, *Musca domestica* L., *J. Insect Physiol.,* 13, 219, 1967.

90. **Dutky, R. C., Robbins, W. E., Kaplanis, J. N., and Shortino, T. J.,** The sterol esters of housefly eggs, *Comp. Biochem. Physiol.,* 9, 251, 1963.

91. **Lasser, N. L. and Clayton, R. B.,** The intracellular distribution of sterols in *Eurycotis floridana* and its possible relation to subcellular membrane structures, *J. Lipid Res.,* 7, 413, 1966.

92. **Dwivedy, A. K.,** Effect of dietary cholesterol deficiency upon its distribution in the larvae of the housefly, *Musca domestica, J. Insect Physiol.,* 22, 1093, 1976.

93. **Cmelik, S.,** Sterols in the diet and various organs of the caterpillars of the Mopani moth, *Gonimbrasia belina, Z. Physiol. Chem.,* 351, 365, 1970.

94. **Svoboda, J. A., Thompson, M. J., Elden, T. C., and Robbins, W. E.,** Unusual composition of sterols in a phytophagous insect, Mexican bean beetle reared on soybean plants, *Lipids,* 9, 752, 1974.

95. **Svoboda, J. A., Thompson, M. J., Robbins, W. E., and Elden, T. C.,** Unique pathways of sterol metabolism in the Mexican bean beetle, a plant feeding insect, *Lipids,* 10, 524, 1975.

95a. **Svoboda, J. A. and Robbins, W. E.,** Comparison of sterols from a phytophagous and predacious species of the family Coccinellidae, *Experientia,* 35, 186, 1979.

96. **Robbins, W. E. and Shortino, T. J.,** Effect of cholesterol in the larval diet on ovarian development in the adult house fly, *Nature,* 194, 502, 1962.

97. **Monroe, R. E., Kaplanis, J. N., and Robbins, W. E.,** Sterol storage and reproduction in the house fly, *Ann. Ent. Soc. Am.,* 54, 537, 1961.

98. **Robbins, W. E., Thompson, M. J., Kaplanis, J. N., and Shortino, T. J.,** The conversion of cholesterol to 7-dehydrocholesterol in asceptically reared German cockroaches, *Steroids,* 4, 635, 1964.

99. **Monroe, R. E.,** Metabolism and utilization of cholesterol-4-C^{14} for growth and reproduction of asceptically-reared house flies, *Musca domestica* L., Ph.D. thesis, Kansas State University, 1964; University Microfilms, Inc., Ann Arbor, Mich., 64-9995, 1965.

99a. **Sang, J. H. and King, R. C.,** Nutritional requirements of axenically cultured *Drosphila melanogaster* adults, *J. Exptl. Biol.,* 38, 793, 1961.

100. **Monroe, R. E.,** Effect of dietary cholesterol on housefly reproduction, *Ann. Ent. Soc. Am.,* 53, 821, 1960.

101. **Svoboda, J. A., Thompson, M. J., and Robbins, W. E.,** 3β-Hydroxy-24-norchol-5-en-23-oic acid-a new inhibitor of the Δ^{24}-sterol reductase enzyme system(s) in the tobacco hornworm, *Steroids,* 12, 559, 1968.

102. **Smissman, E. E., Jenny, N. A., and Beck, S. D.,** Sterol metabolism in the confused flour beetle, *Tribolium confusum, J. Pharm. Sci.,* 53, 1515, 1964.

103. **Pasteels, J. M. and Daloze, D.,** Cardiac glycosides in the defensive secretion of crysomelid beetles: evidence for their production by insects, *Science,* 197, 70, 1977.

104. **Brower, L. P., Brower, J. V. Z., and Corvino, J. M.,** Plant poisons in a terrestrial food chain, *Proc. Nat. Acad. Sci.,* 57, 893, 1967.

105. **Brower, L. P., Ryerson, W. N., Coppinger, L. L., and Glazier, S. C.,** Ecological chemistry and the palatability spectrum, *Science,* 161, 1349, 1968.

106. **Campbell, B. C. and Duffey, S. S.,** Tomatine and parasitic wasps: Potential incompatability of plant antibiosis with biological control, *Science,* 205, 700, 1979.

107. **Bade, M. L. and Clayton, R. B.,** Cholesterol esters of the cockroach *Eurycotis floridana, Nature,* 197, 77, 1963.

108. **Hutchins, R. F. N. and Kaplanis, J. N.,** Sterol sulfates in an insect, *Steroids,* 13, 605, 1969.

109. **Frantz, I. D., Jr., Sanghvi, A. J., and Schroepfer, G. J.,** Irreversibility of the biosynthetic sequence from Δ^7-cholesten-3β-ol through $\Delta^{5,7}$-cholestadien-3β-ol to cholesterol, *J. Biol. Chem.,* 239, 1007, 1964.

110. **Kaplanis, J. N., Monroe, R. E., Robbins, W. E., and Louloudes, S. J.,** The fate of dietary ^{3}H-sitosterol in the adult house fly, *Ann. Ent. Soc. Am.,* 56, 198, 1963.

111. **Clayton, R. B. and Edwards, A. M.,** Conversion of 5α-cholestan-3β-ol to Δ^7-5α-cholesten-3β-ol in cockroaches, *J. Biol. Chem.,* 238, 1966, 1963.

112. **Chapman, J. C., Lockley, W. J. S., Rees, H. H., and Goodwin, T. W.,** Stereochemistry of olefinic bond formation in defensive secretions of *Acilius sulcatus* (Dysticidae), *Eur. J. Biochem.,* 81, 293, 1977.

113. **Svoboda, J. A., Womack, M., Thompson, M. J.,and Robbins, W. E.,** Comparative studies on the activity of 3β-hydroxy-Δ^5-norcholenic acid on the Δ^{24}-sterol reductase enzyme(s) in an insect and the rat, *Comp. Biochem. Physiol.,* 30, 541, 1969.

114. **Svoboda, J. A. and Robbins, W. E.,** The inhibitive effects of azasterols on sterol metabolism and growth and development in insects with special reference to the tobacco hornworm, *Lipids,* 6, 113, 1971.

115. **Wientjens, W. H. J. M., van der Marel, T., and Bennett, E. P.,** The influence of several steroids on the conversion of β-sitosterol into cholesterol in the cockroach, *Experientia,* 27, 373, 1971.

116. **Pettler, P. J., Lockley, W. J. S., Rees, H. H., and Goodwin, T. W.,** Migration of the C_{25} hydrogen of clionasterol to the C_{24} position during dealkylation by the insect *Tenebrio molitor, J. Chem. Soc., Chem. Comm.,* 844, 1974.

117. **Thompson, M. J., Svoboda, J. A., Kaplanis, J. N., and Robbins, W. E.,** Metabolic pathways of steroids in insects, *Proc. R. Soc. London Ser. B,* 180, 203, 1972.

118. **Robbins, W. E., Dutky, R. C., Monroe, R. E., and Kaplanis, J. N.,** The metabolism of ^{3}H-β-sitosterol by the German cockroach, *Ann. Ent. Soc. Am.,* 55, 102, 1962.

119. **Schaefer, C. H. S., Kaplanis, J. N., and Robbins, W. E.,** The relationship of the sterols of the Virginia pine sawfly, *Neodiprion pratti* Dyar, to those of two host plants, *Pinus virginia* Mill and *Pinus rigida* Mill, *J. Insect. Physiol.,* 11, 1013, 1965.

120. **Ikekawa, N., Suzuki, M., Kobayashi, M., and Tsuda, K.,** Dealkylation of sitosterol to cholesterol in the silkworm, *Bombyx mori, Chem. Pharm. Bull.,* 14, 834, 1966.

121. **Allais, J. P., Pain, J., and Barbier, M.,** Dealkylation at C_{24} of β-sitosterol by the bee, *Apis mellifica, Compt. Rend. D,* 272, 877, 1971.

122. **Jackson, L. L., Baker, G. L., and Henry, J. E.,** Effect of *Malamoeba locustae* infection on the egg lipids of the grasshopper *Melanoplus bivittatus, J. Insect Physiol.,* 14, 1773, 1968.

123. **Martin, M. M. and Carls, G. A.,** The lipids of the common house cricket, *Acheta domesticus* L., III. Sterols, *Lipids,* 3, 256, 1968.

124. **Svoboda, J. A., Thompson, M. J., and Robbins, W. E.,** Identification of fucosterol as a metabolite and probable intermediate in conversion of β-sitosterol to cholesterol in the tobacco hornworm, *Nature, N. Biol.,* 230, 57, 1971.

125. **Allais, J. P. and Barbier, M.,** Intermediates in the dealkylation of β-sitosterol by the locust, *Locusta migratoria, Experientia,* 27, 506, 1971.

126. **Ikekawa, N., Morisaki, M., Ohtaka, H., and Chiyoda, Y.,** Reaction of fucosterol epoxide with boron trifluoride etherate, *J. Chem. Soc. Chem. Comm.,* 1468, 1971; Ohtaka, H., Morisaki, M., and Ikekawa, N., Reaction of 24,28-epoxides of sterol side chain with boron trifluoride etherate, *J. Org. Chem.,* 38, 1688, 1973.

127. **Allais, J. P., Alcaide, A., and Barbier, M.,** Fucosterol 24,28-epoxide and 28-oxo-β-sitosterol as possible intermediates in the conversion of β-sitosterol into cholesterol in the locust, *Locusta migratoria* L., *Experientia,* 29, 944, 1973.

128. **Randall, P. J., Lloyd-Jones, J. G., Cook, I. F., Rees, H. H., and Goodwin, T. W.,** The fate of the C_{25} hydrogen of 28-isofucosterol during conversion of this into cholesterol in the insect *Tenebrio molitor, J. Chem. Soc., Chem. Comm.,* 1296, 1972.

129. **Pettler, P. J., Lockley, W. J. S., Rees, H. H., and Goodwin, T. W.,** Mechanism of dealkylation of clionasterol in the insect *Tenebrio molitor, Biochem. J.,* 174, 397, 1979.

130. **Fujimoto, Y., Awata, N., Morisaki, M., and Ikekawa, N.,** Migration of C-25 hydrogen of sitosterol to C-24 during the conversion into desmosterol in the silkworm *Bombyx mori, Tet. Lett.,* 4335, 1974.

131. **Chen, S.-M., Nakanishi, K., Awata, N., Morisaki, M., Ikekawa, N., and Shimizu, Y.,** Stereospecificity in the conversion of fucosterol 24,28-epoxide to desmosterol in the silkworm, *Bombyx mori, J. Am. Chem. Soc.,* 97, 5297, 1975.

131a. **Fujimoto, Y., Murakami, K., and Ikekawa, N.,** Synthesis of (24R,28R)- and (24S,28S)-fucosterol epoxides. Revision of $C_{24,28}$ configurations, *J. Org. Chem.,* 45, 566, 1980.

131b. **Fujimoto, Y., Morisaki, M., and Ikekawa, N.,** Stereochemical importance of fucosterol epoxide in the conversion of sitosterol into cholesterol in the silkworm, *Bombyx mori, Biochemistry,* 19, 1065, 1980.

131c. **Nicotra, F., Ronchetti, F., Russo, G., and Toma, L.,** Conversion of isofucosterol-(24R,28S)-epoxide into cholesterol in the insect *Tenebrio molitor, J. Chem. Soc. Chem. Comm.,* 479, 1980.

131d. **Morisaki, M., Ying, B., and Ikekawa, N.,** Identification of both fucosterol and isofucosterol in the silkworm, *Bombyx mori, Experientia,* 37, 336, 1981.

132. **Awata, N., Morisaki, M., and Ikekawa, N.,** Carbon-carbon bond cleavage of fucosterol 24,28-epoxide by cell-free extracts of the silkworm, *Bombyx mori, Biochem. Biophys. Res. Comm.,* 44, 157, 1975.

133. **Awata, N., Morisaki, M., Fujimoto, Y., and Ikekawa, N.,** Inhibitory effects of steroidal allenes on growth, development, and steroid metabolism of the silkworm, *Bombyx mori, J. Insect Physiol.,* 22, 403, 1976.

134. **Kaplanis, J. N., Dutky, S. R., Robbins, W. E., Thompson, M. J., Lindquist, E. L., Horn, D. H. S., and Galbraith, M. N.,** Makisterone A: A 28-carbon hexahydroxy molting hormone from the embryo of the milkweed bug, *Science,* 190, 681, 1975.

135. **Goetz, M., Wiemer, D. F., Haynes, L. R. W., Meinwald, J., and Eisner, T.,** Lucibufagines Partie III. Oxo-11 et oxo-12-bufalines, steroides difensifs des lampyres *Photius ignitus* et *P. marginellus, Helv. Chim. Acta,* 62, 1396, 1979.

136. **Essig, E. O.,** How insects live, in *Insects, The Yearbook of Agriculture,* U.S. Dept. Agric., Washington, D.C., 1954, 24.

137. **Babers, F. H. and Pratt, J. J., Jr.,** Life processes of insects, in *Insects, The Yearbook of Agriculture,* U.S. Dept. Agric., Washington, D.C., 1954, 30.

138. **Gilbert, L. I. and King, D. S.,** Physiology of growth and development: endocrine aspects, in *The Physiology of Insects,* Vol. 1, 2nd ed., Rockstein, M., Ed., Academic Press, New York, 1973, chap. 5.

139. **Gilbert, L. I., Goodman, W., and Bollenbacker, W. E.,** Biochemistry of regulatory lipids and sterols in insects, in *Biochemistry of Lipids II. International Review of Biochemistry,* Vol. 14, Goodwin, T. W., Ed., University Park Press, Baltimore, 1977, chap. 1.

140. **Butenandt, A. and Karlson, P.,** Uber die Isolierung eines Metamorphose-Hormons der Insekten in Kristalli-sierter Form, *Z. Naturforsh.,* 9b, 389, 1954.

141. **Karlson, P., Hoffmeister, H., Hoppe, W., and Huber, R.,** Zur Chemie des Ecdysons, I. *Leibigs Ann.,* 662, 1, 1963; II-VII. *Chem. Ber.,* 98, 2353-2403, 1965.

142. **Siddall, J. B., Cross, A. D., and Fried, J. H.,** Steroids CCXCII. Synthetic studies on insect hormones. II. The synthesis of ecdysone, *J. Am. Chem. Soc.,* 88, 862, 1966.

143. **Kerb, U., Hocks, P., and Weichert, R.,** The synthesis of ecdysone, Tet. Letters, 13, 1387, 1966, *Helv. Chim. Acta,* 49; 1581, 1591, 1601; 1966.

144. **Dahm, K. H., Trost, B. M., and Roller, H.,** The juvenile hormone. V. Synthesis of the racemic juvenile hormone, *J. Am. Chem. Soc.,* 89, 5292, 1967.

145. **Hampshire, F. and Horn, D. H. S.,** Structure of crustecdysone, a crustacean molting hormone, *Chem. Comm.,* 37, 1966.

146. **Kaplanis, J. N., Robbins, W. E., Thompson, M. J., and Dutky, S. R.,** 26-Hydroxyecdysone, a new insect molting hormone from the egg of the tobacco hornworm, *Science,* 180, 307, 1973.

147. **Ohnishi, E., Mizuno, T., Chatani, F., Ikekawa, N., and Sakurai, S.,** 2-Deoxyecdysone from ovaries and eggs of the silkworm, *Bombyx mori, Science,* 197, 66, 1977.

147a. **Dinan, L. N. and Rees, H. H.,** The identification and titres of conjugated and free ecdysteroids in developing ovaries and newly laid eggs of *Schistocerca gregaria, J. Insect Physiol.,* 27, 51, 1981.

148. **Robbins, W. E., Kaplanis, J. N., Svoboda, J. A., and Thompson, M. J.,** Steroid metabolism in insects, *Ann. Rev. Entomol.,* 16, 53, 1971.

149. **Cook, I. F., Lloyd-Jones, J. G., Rees, H. H., and Goodwin, T. W.,** The stereochemistry of hydrogen elimination from C-7 during biosynthesis of ecdysones in insects and plants, *Biochem. J.,* 136, 135, 1973.

149a. **Davis, T. G., Dinan, L. N., Lockley, W. J. S., Rees, H. H., and Goodwin, T. W.,** Formation of A/B *cis* ring junction of ecdysteroids in the locust *Schistocerca gregaria, Biochem. J.,* 194, 53, 1981.

150. **Johnson, P. and Rees, H.,** Biosynthesis of ecdysones: Metabolism of 7-dehydrocholesterol in *Schistocerca, J. Insect Physiol.,* 23, 1387, 1977.

151. **Galbraith, M. N., Horn, D. H. S., Middleton, E. J., Thomson, J. A., and Wilkie, J. S.,** Metabolism of $3\beta,14\alpha$-dihydroxy-5β-(3α-^{3}H)-cholest-7-en-6-one in *Calliphora stygia, J. Insect Physiol.,* 21, 23, 1975.

152. **Svoboda, J. A., Kaplanis, J. N., Robbins, W. E., and Thompson, M. J.,** Recent developments in insect steroid metabolism, *Ann. Rev. Entomol.,* 20, 205, 1975.

152a. **Smith, S. L., Bollenbacher, W. E., Cooper, D. Y., Schleyer, H., Wielgus, J. J., and Gilbert, L. I.,** Ecdysone 20-monooxygenase: Characterization of an insect cytochrome P-450 dependent steroid hydroxylase, *Mol. and Cell. Endocrinol.*, 15, 111, 1979.

153. **Sakurai, S., Ikekawa, N., Ohtaki, T., and Chino, H.,** 3β-Hydroxy-5α-cholestan-6-one: A possible precursor of α-ecdysone biosynthesis, *Science*, 198, 627, 1977.

154. **Kinnear, J. F., Martin, M.-D., Chong, Y. K., Faux, A., Horn, D. H. S., and Wilkie, J. S.,** Insect molting hormones: Possible intermediates in the metabolism of cholesterol to ecdysteroids, *Aust. J. Chem.*, 31, 2069, 1978.

155. **Faux, A. F., Horn, D. H. S., Kinnear, J. F., Martin, M.-D., Wilkie, J. S., and Willing, R. I.,** Evaluation of 3β-hydroxy-5β-cholest-7-en-6-one and related steroids as precursors of ecdysteroids in *Calliphora stygia, Insect Biochem.*, 9, 101, 1979.

156. **Romer, F., Emmerich, H., and Nowock, J.,** Biosynthesis of ecdysones in isolated prothoracic glands and oenocytes of *Tenebrio molitor* in vitro, *J. Insect Physiol.*, 20, 1975, 1974.

157. **Willig, A., Rees, H. H., and Goodwin, T. W.,** Biosynthesis of insect molting hormones in isolated ring glands and whole larvae of *Calliphora, J. Insect Physiol.*, 17, 2317, 1971.

158. **Gersch, M. and Sturzebecker, J.,** Synthesis of ^{3}H-ecdysone from ^{3}H-cholesterol in ligated abdomens of *Mamestra brassicae* larvae, *Experientia*, 27, 1475, 1971.

159. **Nakanishi, K., Moriyama, H., Okauchi, T., Fujioka, S., and Koreeda, M.,** Biosynthesis of α- and β-ecdysones from cholesterol outside the prothoracic gland in *Bombyx mori, Science*, 176, 51, 1972.

160. **Lafont, R., Mauchamp, B., Pennetier, J-L., and DeReggi, M. L.,** Endocrine significance of critical periods during insect development: Analysis of ligation experiments with *Pieris brassicae* last instar larvae, *Experientia*, 33, 1662, 1977.

161. **Legay, J. M., Calvez, B., Hirn, M., and DeReggi, M. L.,** Ecdysone and oocyte morphogenesis in *Bombyx mori, Nature*, 262, 489, 1976.

162. **Garen, A., Kauvar, L., and Lepesant, J-A.,** Roles of ecdysone in *Drosophila* development, *Proc. Nat. Acad. Sci.*, 74, 5099, 1977.

163. **Lagueux, M., Hirn, M., and Hoffmann, J. A.,** Ecdysone during ovarian development in *Locusta migratoria, J. Insect Physiol.*, 23, 109, 1977.

164. **Charlet, M., Goltzene, F., and Hoffman, J. A.,** Experimental evidence for neuroendocrine control of ecdysone biosynthesis in adult females of *Locusta migratoria, J. Insect Physiol.*, 25, 463, 1979.

164a. **Hagedorn, H. H., Shapiro, J. P., and Hanaoka, K.,** Ovarian ecdysone secretion is controlled by a brain hormone in an adult mosquito, *Nature (London)*, 282, 92, 1979.

165. **Delbeque, J.-P. A., Delachambre, J., Hirn, M., and de Reggi, M.,** Abdominal production of ecdysterone and pupal-adult development in *Tenebrio molitor* (Insecta: Coleoptera), *Gen. and Comp. Endocrinol.*, 35, 436, 1978.

166. **Sekeris, C. E. and Karlson, P.,** On the mechanism of hormone action. II. Ecdysone and protein synthesis, *Arch. Biochem. Biophys.*, 105, 483, 1964.

167. **Sekeris, C. E., Lang, N., and Karlson, P.,** Influence of ecdysone on RNA turnover in the epidermis of the fly *Calliphora erythrocephala, Z. fur Physiol. Chem.*, 341, 36, 1965.

168. **Sekeris, C. E., Dukes, P. P., and Schmid, W.,** Action of ecdysone on epidermal cell nuclei of *Calliphora*-larvae in vitro, *Z. fur Physiol. Chem.*, 341, 152, 1965.

169. **Scheller, K. and Karlson, P.,** Effect of ecdysteroids on RNA synthesis of fat body cells in *Calliphora vicina, J. Insect Physiol.*, 23, 285, 1977.

170. **Valentin, M., Bollenbacker, W. E., Gilbert, L. I., and Kroeger, H.,** Alterations in ecdysone content during the post-embryonic development of *Chironomus thummi*: Correlations with chromosome puffing, *Zeit. fur Naturforsch.*, 33c, 557, 1978.

171. **Johnson, P. and Rees, H. H.,** The mechanism of C-20-hydroxylation of α-ecdysone in the desert locust, *Schistocerca gregaria, Biochem. J.*, 168, 513, 1977.

172. **Yund, M. A.,** Ecdysteroid action in imaginal discs of *Drosophila melanogaster* does not involve cyclic AMP, *J. Insect Physiol.*, 25, 781, 1979.

173. **Beach, R.,** Mosquitos: Biting behavior inhibited by ecdysone, *Science*, 205, 829, 1979.

174. **Kaplanis, J. N., Tabor, L. A., Thompson, M. J., Robbins, W. E., and Shortino, T. J.,** Assay for ecdysone (molting hormone) activity using the housefly, *Musca domestica* L., *Steroids*, 8, 625, 1966.

175. **Ohtaki, T., Milkman, R. D., and Williams, C. M.,** Ecdysone and ecdysone analogs; their assay on the fleshfly, *Sarcophaga peregrina, Proc. Natl. Acad. Sci.*, 58, 981, 1967.

176. **Robbins, W. E., Kaplanis, J. N., Thompson, M. J., Shortino, T. J., and Joyner, S. C.,** Ecdysones and synthetic analogs. Moulting hormone activity and inhibitive effects on insect growth, metamorphosis and reproduction, *Steroids*, 16, 105, 1970.

176a. **Singh, P. and Russell, G. B.,** The dietary effects of 20-hydroxyecdysone on the development of the house fly, *J. Insect Physiol.*, 26, 139, 1980.

177. **Rees, H. H.,** Ecdysones, in *Aspects of Terpenoid Chemistry and Biochemistry*, Goodwin, T. W., Ed., Academic Press, London, 1971, Chap. 7.

178. **Hora, J., Labler, L., Kasal, A., Cerny, V., and Sorm, F.,** Moulting deficiencies produced by some sterol derivatives in an insect (*Pyrrhocoris apterus* L.), *Steroids,* 8, 887, 1966.

179. **Sroka, P. and Gilbert, L. I.,** Studies on the endocrine control of post-emergence ovarian maturation in *Manduca sexta, J. Insect Physiol.,* 17, 2409, 1971.

180. **Sakurai, H.,** Endocrine control of oogenesis in the housefly, *Musca domestica vicina, J. Insect Physiol.,* 23, 1295, 1977.

181. **Hagedorn, H. H., Turner, S., Hagedorn, E. A., Pontecorvo, D., Greenbaum, P., Pfeiffer, D., Wheelock, G., and Flanagan, T. R.,** Postemergence growth of the ovarian follicles of *Aedes aegypti, J. Insect Physiol.,* 23, 203, 1977.

182. **Luscher, M.,** Hormonal control of respiration and protein synthesis in the fat body of the cockroach *Nauphoeta cinerea* during oocyte growth, *J. Insect Physiol.,* 14, 499, 1968.

183. **Engelmann, F.,** Female specific protein: Biosynthesis controlled by corpus allatum in *Leucophaea maderae, Science,* 165, 407, 1969.

184. **Pan, M. L. and Wyatt, G. R.,** Juvenile hormone induces vitellogenin synthesis in the monarch butterfly, *Science,* 174, 503, 1971.

185. **Spielman, A., Gwadz, R. W., and Anderson, W. A.,** Ecdysone initiated ovarian development in mosquitoes, *J. Insect Physiol.,* 17, 1807, 1971.

186. **Hetru, C., Lagueux, M., Bang, L., and Hoffman, J. A.,** Adult ovaries of *Locusta migratoria* contain the sequence of biosynthetic intermediates for ecdysone, *Life Sci.,* 22, 2141, 1978.

187. **Postlethwait, J. H. and Handler, A. M.,** The roles of juvenile hormone and 20-hydroxyecdysone during vitellogenesis in isolated abdomens of *Drosophila melanogaster, J. Insect Physiol.,* 25, 455, 1979.

187a. **Stay, B., Friedel, T., Tobe, S. S., and Mundall, E. C.,** Feedback control of juvenile hormone synthesis in cockroaches: Possible role for ecdysterone, *Science,* 207, 898, 1980.

188. **Wright, J. E., Chamberlain, W. F., and Barrett, C. C.,** Ovarian maturation in stable flies: Inhibition by 20-hydroxyecdysone, *Science,* 172, 1247, 1971.

189. **Garcia, M. L. M., Mello, R. P., and Garcia, E. S.,** Ecdysone, juvenile hormone and oogenesis in *Rodnius prolixus, J. Insect Physiol.,* 25, 695, 1979.

190. **Kambysellis, M. P. and Williams, C. M.,** Spermatogenesis in cultured testes of the cynthia silkworm: Effects of ecdysone and prothoracic glands, *Science,* 175, 769, 1972.

191. **Hoffmeister, H., Rufer, C., and Ammon, H.,** Excretion of ecdysone by insects, *Z. fur Naturforsch.,* 20b, 130, 1965.

192. **Greenwood, D. R. and Russell, G. B.,** 26-Hydroxyecdysone, a metabolite of β-ecdysone in the blowfly, *Calliphora erythrocephala, Experientia,* 34, 687, 1978.

193. **Nigg, H. N., Svoboda, J. A., Thompson, M. J., Kaplanis, J. N., Dutky, S. R., and Robbins, W. E.,** Ecdysone metabolism: Ecdysone dehydrogenase-isomerase, *Lipids,* 9, 971, 1974.

194. **Koolman, J. and Karlson, P.,** Ecdysone oxidase: Reaction and specificity, *Eur. J. Biochem.,* 89, 453, 1978.

195. **Galbraith, M. N. and Horn, D. H. S.,** An insect molting hormone from a plant, *Chem. Comm.,* 905, 1966.

196. **Nakanishi, K., Koreeda, M., Sasaki, S., Chang, M. L., and Hsu, H. Y.,** Insect hormones, the structure of Ponasterone A, an insect moulting hormone from leaves of *Podocarpus nakaii* Hay., *Chem. Comm.,* 915, 1966.

197. **Carlisle, D. B. and Ellis, P. E.,** Bracken and locust ecdysones: their effects on moulting in the desert locust, *Science,* 159, 1472, 1968.

198. **Sauer, H. H., Bennett, R. D., and Heftmann, E.,** Ecdysone biosynthesis in *Podocarpus elata, Phytochem.,* 7, 2027, 1968.

199. **Schneiderman, H. A., Krishnakumaran, A., Bryant, P. J., and Sehnal, F.,** Endocrinological strategies in insect control, *Agric. Sci. Rev.,* 2nd and 3rd Qtr. 1970.

Chapter 2

CHOLESTEROL AND MEMBRANES

Rosemarie Ostwald

TABLE OF CONTENTS

I. INTRODUCTION

In this chapter I have attempted to outline for nonmembrane specialists the presently most widely accepted concepts concerning the structure of biological membranes, the spatial distribution of their components, and the role(s) played by the lipids in some of their major functions with emphasis on the function of cholesterol.

I did not intend to present a comprehensive review of the present state of information in this field. Therefore, much of the information I have used has previously been reviewed (see References 1 to 6). I did add some of the work from my own laboratory and some recent literature of specific interest to me.

In most instances I have touched only lightly on the details of the experimental evidence for a particular statement. Interested readers will find these details in the literature cited.

II. MEMBRANE FUNCTIONS

Biological membranes are the structures that surround all living cells and most subcellular units, such as mitochondria, endoplasmic reticulum, golgi apparatus, nuclei, and lysosomes. They function to maintain the compositional differences between two aqueous compartments such as the inside and outside of a cell, or to permit change in a controlled manner. They were previously thought to be inert packaging materials, but are now known to fulfill a multitude of functions and to have a rather complicated structure.

Membranes serve as screens to permit entry to and exit from the cell or compartment of nutrients and metabolic products where the screen can be either a passive barrier or an active transport system; they are the origins and carriers of electrical impulses in excitable membranes such as nerve axons; they function as energy transducers in membranes of photosynthetic organisms and visual systems; and they carry structures responsible for the recognition of substances regulating cell metabolism such as hormones and plasma lipoproteins as well as for cell-cell recognition that are essential for morphogenesis, immune responses, and carcinogenesis. Considering this variety of functions, composition and structure of membranes of different origins are remarkably similar.

III. MEMBRANE COMPOSITION

Lipids and proteins are quantitatively the major components but their relative amounts differ in different membrane systems (Table 1). The more metabolically active the system, the higher is the protein to lipid ratio. For instance, the major component of myelin that functions primarily as electrical insulator is lipid. Most cell membranes of animals serving predominantly transport functions contain approximately equal amounts of proteins and lipids. Plasma membranes of bacterial cells and of inner membranes of mitochondria that are associated with oxidative phosphorylation and synthesis of nucleic acids contain up to two thirds of their mass as protein. Most membranes also contain small, but functionally very important, amounts of carbohydrates.

The isolation, separation, and characterization of membrane proteins and their polypeptide chains is presently an area of intense study but beyond the scope of this essay.[7]

The major lipids in membranes are phospholipids and sterols. Small amounts of other compounds such as carotenoids, tocopherols, and quinones have been reported in some membranes.[8] They perform essential functions in these specialized membranes but will not be considered here further.

Table 1
COMPOSITION OF CELL MEMBRANES

Membrane	Protein %	Lipid, %	Carbohydrate, %	Weight fraction of protein	Ratio of protein to lipid
Myelin	18	79	3	0.18	0.23
Plasma membranes					
Blood platelets	33—42	58—51	7.5	0.4	0.7
Mouse liver cells	46	54	2—4	0.46	0.85
Human erythrocyte	49	43	8	0.49	1.1
Amoeba	54	42	4	0.54	1.3
Rat liver cells	58	42	(5-10)	0.58	1.4
Nuclear membrane of rat liver cells	59	35	2.9	0.59	1.6
Retinal rods, bovine	51	49	4	0.51	1.0
Mitochondrial outer membrane	52	48	(2-4)	0.52	1.1
Sarcoplasmic reticulum	67	33		0.67	2.0
Mitochondrial inner membrane	76	24	(1-2)	0.76	3.2
Gram-positive bacteria	75	25	(10)	0.75	3.0
Halobacterium purple membrane	75	25		0.75	3.0
Mycoplasma	58	37	1.5	0.58	1.6

From Chapman, D. ,*Mammalian Cell Membranes,* Jamieson, G. and Robinson, D., Eds., Vol. 1, Butterworth, London, 1976. With permission.

A. Phospholipids

The main classes of membrane phospholipids are phosphatidylcholine (lecithin, PC), phosphatidylethanolamine (PE), phosphatidylserine (PS), phosphatidylinositol (PI), and sphingomyelin. Cardiolipin (diphosphatidylglycerol), the characteristic phospholipid of the inner mitochondrial membrane, is present in smaller amounts in some other membranes as well. The first four, derivatives of phosphatidic acid, carry two fatty acyl chains. Sphingomyelin also has two hydrocarbon chains, one from the sphingosine base, the other an acyl chain as amide of the amino group (Figure 1). Some membranes, especially myelin, contain appreciable amounts of galactolipids (often called glycolipids or cerebrosides), gangliosides, and sulfatides.

The major fatty acids are those with 16 and 18 carbon atoms and zero to two double bonds. Appreciable amounts of longer chain, highly unsaturated fatty acids also occur in certain membranes.

The possible combinations of different polar head groups, and of different fatty acids in the two possible positions and in different linkages to the glycerol backbone (ester, vinyl ether, or ether bonds), permit an almost infinite variety in the composition of a membrane and therefore in functional parameters. The proportions of both phospholipid head groups and individual fatty acids is rather different for different types of membranes but are in a general way characteristic for a given membrane in different tissues and for a given membrane type in different animal species. The distribution of the different phospholipids and their constituent fatty acids in a large variety of membranes has been studied in detail (Reference 5, Volume 1, Chapters 5, 9, and 10) and will be covered here only to the extent necessary for the discussion of the functions of cholesterol.

B. Cholesterol

Cholesterol (cholest-5-en-3β-ol) is the major sterol in animal membranes. Some closely related sterols such as 7-dehydrocholesterol and desmosterol have also been detected. Stigmasterol, sitosterol, and ergosterol are typical sterols found in plants.

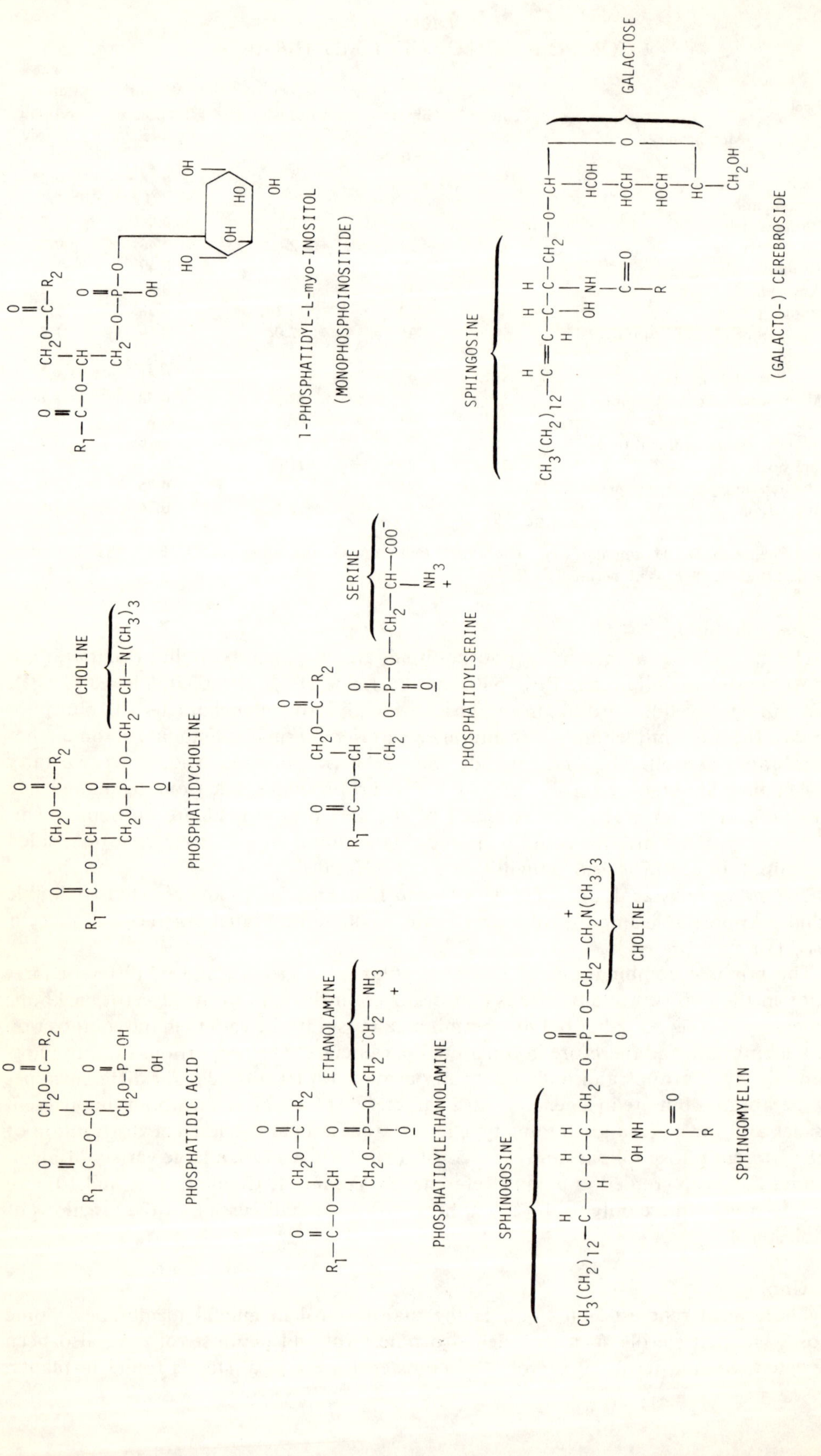

PHOSPHATIDIC ACID

CHOLINE

PHOSPHATIDYCHOLINE

1-PHOSPHATIDYL-L-myo-INOSITOL

(MONOPHOSPHOINOSITIDE)

ETHANOLAMINE

PHOSPHATIDYLETHANOLAMINE

SERINE

PHOSPHATIDYLSERINE

SPHINOGOSINE

CHOLINE

SPHINGOMYELIN

SPHINGOSINE

GALACTOSE

(GALACTO-) CEREBROSIDE

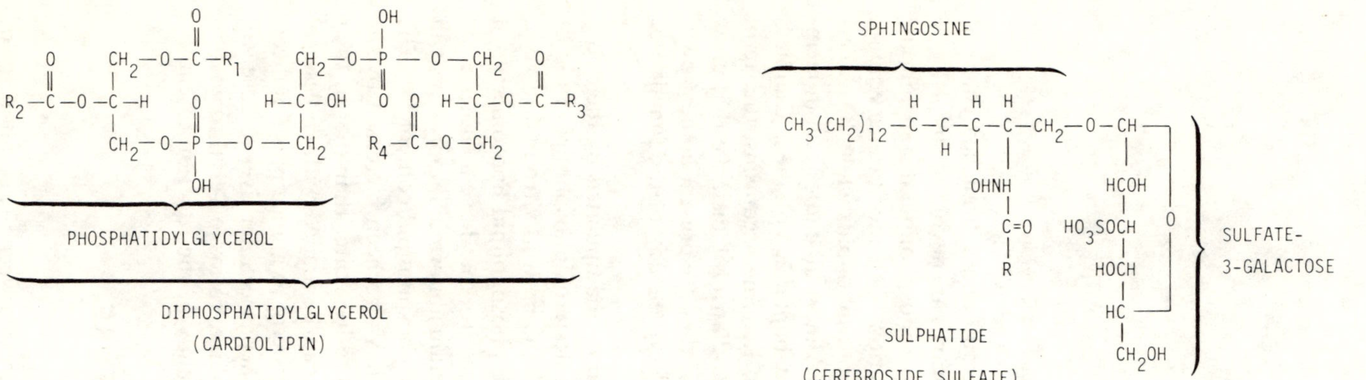

FIGURE 1. Structures of some phospholipids important as membrane constituents.

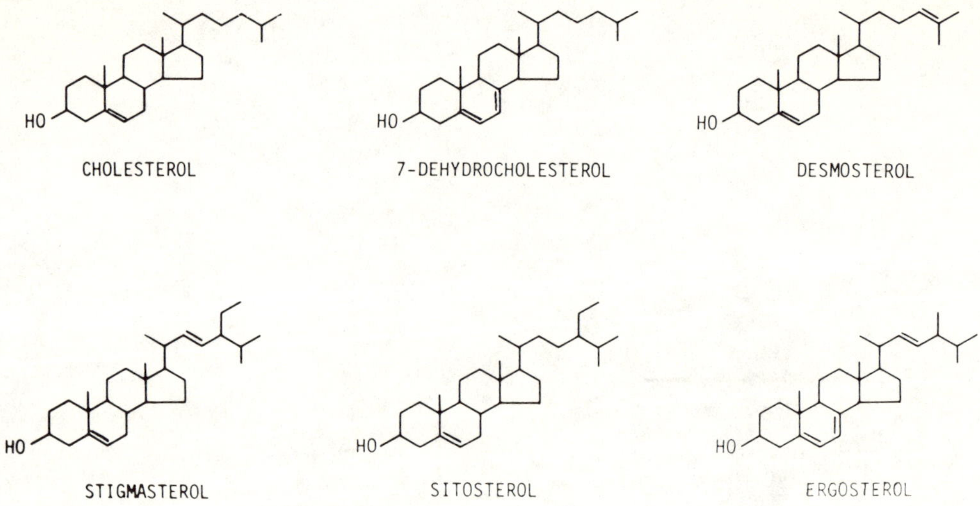

CHOLESTEROL 7-DEHYDROCHOLESTEROL DESMOSTEROL

STIGMASTEROL SITOSTEROL ERGOSTEROL

FIGURE 2. Structures of some mammalian and plant sterols.

All of them have a planar sterol nucleus, a 3β-OH group and a branched chain of eight or more carbons at C_{17} (Figure 2). Bacterial membranes are devoid of sterols.

The amount of cholesterol and the ratio of cholesterol/phospholipid in a membrane relates to its barrier rather than to its metabolic function. Cell membranes contain approximately equal molar amounts of cholesterol and phospholipids while the cholesterol content of subcellular membranes is much lower. Almost all cholesterol in membranes is unesterified (Table 2) (Reference 5, Volume 1, Chapter 2; Volume 2, Chapters 1 and 7; Volume 3, Chapter 1; Volume 4, Chapter 10). In some organisms, the sterol content of membranes can be varied. *Acholeplasma laidlawii* for instance that grow in the absence of sterols will incorporate several sterols if they are present in the growth medium.[11] Consequently, this organism is very useful for the study of the function of different sterols in membranes.

The cholesterol content of some microorganisms can be manipulated by their conditions of growth.[12] The cholesterol content and the cholesterol/phospholipid ratio of erythrocytes (RBC) can be varied within rather wide limits both in vitro and in vivo. Incubation of RBC with lipid-depleted plasma, or with phospholipid liposomes[13] will decrease their cholesterol content. Incubation with liposomes that have a cholesterol/phospholipid ratio greater than that of RBC or with certain abnormal lipoproteins will increase their cholesterol without much change in their phospholipid content.[14,15] The cholesterol content of certain other mammalian cells has also been increased by the exposure to liposomes with a cholesterol/phospholipid ratio greater than that of their membranes.[16,17] Liver mitochondrial membranes also can be loaded with cholesterol by incubation with certain lipoproteins.[18] Feeding cholesterol to guinea pigs[19] and certain pathological conditions in humans such as severe hepatocellular liver disease will increase cholesterol content and cholesterol/phospholipid ratios of erythrocytes in vivo.[20] Such membranes serve as useful tools for the study of the function of cholesterol.

IV. MEMBRANE STRUCTURE

A. Thermodynamic Considerations

The structure of membranes is determined by the forces between the components of the system. Therefore, any membrane model must be compatible with a minimum free energy state assumed by the membrane components because of their physicochemical interactions.

Table 2
TOTAL CHOLESTEROL, UNESTERIFIED CHOLESTEROL AND CHOLESTEROL/ PHOSPHOLIPID RATIO IN VARIOUS TISSUES AND CELL MEMBRANES

	TC		FC		TC/PL	
		(% TL)	(g/100 g)	(% TL)	(molar)	(weight)
Liver (human)	0.29[a,1]		80[1]			
Muscle (human)	0.1[a,1]		93[1]			
Kidney (human)	0.28[a,1]		90[1]			
Adult brain (various species)	3-5[a,2]					
Lymphocytes (human)		12.5[3]			0.68[3]	
Erythrocytes (various species)	0.6—0.9[b,4]	25[5]		0.6—0.9[4]		
Erythrocytes (human)		27[3]			0.94[4]	0.81[6]
Erythrocytes (rat)	1.0—1.6[a,1]					0.73[7]
Platelets (human)		21[8]				0.49[9]
Myelin (rat)		25[5]				
Liver (rat)						
Rough microsomes		5.5[10]		4.5[10]	0.04[11]	0.06[10]
Golgi fraction		7.5[10]		3.0[10]	0.14[11]	0.14[10]
Plasma membrane						
Liver (rat)		19.5[10]		17.0[10]	0.21[11]	0.34[10]—0.65[6]
Liver (mouse)					0.46[12]	0.80[6]
Smooth muscle (rat)					0.82[12]	
Kidney brush border (rat)					0.46[12]	

[a] g/100 g wet weight.
[b] g/cell (x 10^{-13}).
[c] mg/g packed cells.

Abbreviations: TC, total cholesterol; FC, unesterified cholesterol; TC/PL, total cholesterol to phospholipid ratio; TL, total lipid.

References to data: 1 **Field, H., Swell, L., Schools, P., and Treadwell, C.,** Dynamic aspects of cholesterol metabolism in different areas of the aorta and other tissues in man and their relationship to atherosIcerosis, *Circulation,* 22, 547, 1960.

Table 2 (continued)
TOTAL CHOLESTEROL, UNESTERIFIED CHOLESTEROL AND CHOLESTEROL/ PHOSPHOLIPID RATIO IN VARIOUS TISSUES AND CELL MEMBRANES

2 **Davison, A.,** Brain sterol metabolism, *Adv. Lipid Res.,* 3, 171, 1965.

3 **Gottfried, E.** Lipids of human leucocytes: Relation to cell type, *J. Lipid Res.,* 8, 321, 1967.

4 **Nelson, G.,** Lipid composition and metabolism of erythrocytes, in, *Blood Lipids and Lipoproteins,* Nelson, G., Ed., chap. 7, Wiley, N.Y., 1972.

5 **Nes, W.,** Role of sterols in membranes, *Lipids,* 9, 596, 1974.

6 **Dodge, J. and Philipps, G.,** Composition of phospholipids and of phospholipid fatty acids and aldehydes in human red cells, *J. Lipid Res.,* 8, 667, 1967.

7 **Nelson, G.,** Composition of neutral lipids from erythrocytes of common mammals, *J. Lipid Res.,* 8, 374, 1967.

8 **Marcus, A., Safier, L., and Ulman, H.,** The lipids of human platelets, in, Blood Lipids and Lipoproteins, Nelson, G., Ed., chap. 9, Wiley, N.Y., 1972.

9 **Barber, A. and Jamieson, G.,** Isolation of glycopeptides from low- and high density platelet plasma membranes, *Biochemistry,* 10, 4711, 1971.

10 **van Hoeven, R., Emmelot, P., Krol, J., and Oomen-Meulemans, E.,** Studies on plasma membranes. XXII. Fatty acid profiles of lipid classes in plasma membranes of rat and mouse livers and hepatomas, *Biochim. Biophys. Acta,* 380, 1, 1975.

11 **Keenan, T. and Morre, D.,** Phospholipid class and fatty acid composition of Golgi apparatus isolated from rat liver and comparison with other cell fractions, *Biochemistry,* 9, 19, 1970.

12 **Glick, M.,** Isolation of surface membranes from mammalian cells in, *Mammalian Cell Membranes,* Jamieson, G., and Robinson, D., Eds.), Vol. 1, Chap. 3, Butterworth, London, 1976.

There are four major types of molecular interactions that are important for the consideration of a system in an aqueous environment: hydrophobic, hydrophilic, hydrogen bondng, and electrostatic.

Hydrophobic forces are responsible for the sequestering of nonpolar groups, such as the hydrocarbon chains of fatty acids, and of nonpolar amino acids away from contact with water. They are the result of the higher negative free energy of water when interacting with itself or polar molecules than with nonpolar molecules.[21]

Hydrophilic interactions are then the tendency for ionic and highly polar groups to remain in immediate contact with water rather than with a nonpolar environment. The importance of these forces has been stressed particularly by Singer.[22]

Hydrogen bonding such as occurs in peptide bonds is maximized within a nonpolar medium because it costs free energy not to do so.

Electrostatic interactions will cause charged groups to seek contact with water. They exist between all charged molecular species, whether in membranes or in solution and will not be considered further here.

B. The Fluid-mosaic Model

The most widely accepted membrane model, the fluid-mosaic model of Singer (Figure 3),[23] is that of a lipid bilayer with proteins either spanning the bilayer or partially buried in the outer or inner leaflet of the bilayer; or as Singer puts it, "a two-dimensional solution of globular integral proteins in a fluid solvent of the lipid bilayer". The lipid bilayer is formed by the phospholipids in which the polar ends are directed outward and the apolar ends inward, forming a sheet with two hydrophilic sides and a hydrophobic center. This maximizes the hydrophilic interactions of the polar head groups with water and minimizes the interactions of the nonpolar regions with water, so producing maximum stability for these amphiphilic molecules (Reference 5, Volume 1, Chapter 10). Similar maximization of hydrophilic and hydrophobic interactions is also required for the stabilization of membrane proteins.

This model is compatible with experimental evidence obtained by a variety of methods using both model systems and biological membranes. The older literature concerning this evidence has been critically reviewed most extensively by Stoeckenius.[3] For recent reviews see Reference 5, Volume 1, Chapter 10.

The position of the polar head groups of phospholipids in relation to the lipid bilayer is still under discussion. Most of the experimental evidence for model systems to date would seem to indicate that the phospholipid dipole is predominantly oriented approximately parallel to the bilayer surface rather than to extend out from it.[24]

Cholesterol is thought to be intercalated between the hydrocarbon chains of the phospholipids (Figure 4). The exact position of cholesterol in respect to the phospholipid has not yet been established because of uncertainties concerning the type of bonds between them. Some investigators have suggested hydrogen bonding between the sterol-OH group and the phosphate ester oxygen atoms of the phospholipids[25] while others find the experimental evidence for such interactions unconvincing.[1,24] A plausible model for the arrangement of phosphatidylcholine and cholesterol in bilayer membranes based on a variety of experimental approaches for their interactions has been proposed.[26]

Although interactions of cholesterol, a very hydrophobic lipid, with proteins was thought to be rather unlikely, it has now been shown in model systems that certain myelin proteins have a high affinity for cholesterol.[27] Other evidence such as effects of cholesterol on enzyme activities will be discussed below. From thermodynamic considerations, it would seem likely that cholesterol will not interact as strongly with polyunsaturated fatty acids as with more saturated hydrocarbon chains (Reference 5, Volume 2, Chapter 1). Since the cholesterol molecule is rigid and planar, a saturated

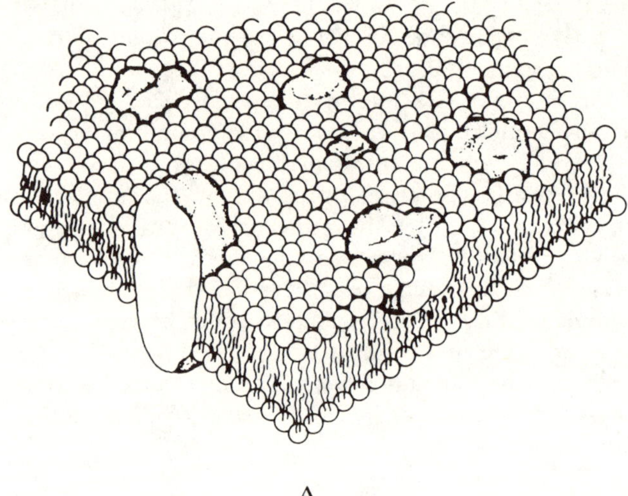

A.

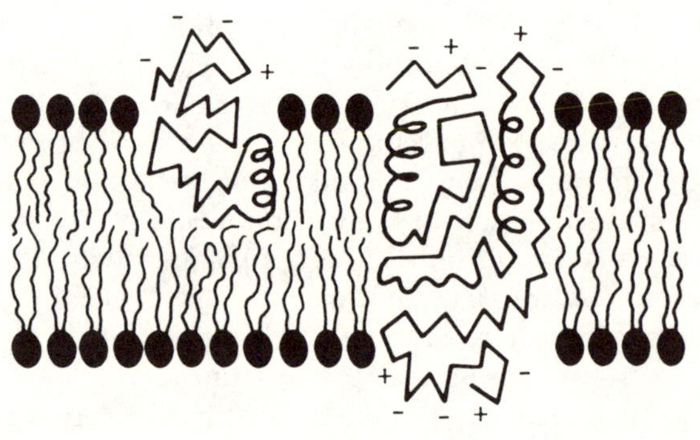

B.

FIGURE 3. The fluid mosaic model of membrane structure. A. Schematic three-dimensional view. The solid bodies with stippled surfaces represent the amphipathic globular integral proteins, embedded in a fluid bilayer of lipid. The circles represent the ionic and polar head groups of the phospholipid molecules; the wavy lines represent the fatty acid chains. (From Singer, S., *Structure and Function of Biological Membranes*, Rothfield, L., Ed., Academic Press, N.Y., 1971, 145. With permission.) B. Schematic cross-sectional view. The phospholipids are arranged as a discontinuous bilayer with their ionic and polar heads in contact with water. The integral proteins, with the heavy lines representing the folded polypeptide chains, are shown as globular molecules partially embedded in, and partially protruding from, the membrane. The protruding parts have on their surfaces the ionic residues (− and +) of the protein, while the nonpolar residues are largely in the embedded parts. (From Singer, S. and Nicolson, G., *Science*, 175, 720, 1972. With permission.)

fatty acid chain would permit closest approach between the molecules and hence maximum effect of binding forces. The oleyl chain (18:1) has a kink but can still be planar like a bent stick that can lie flat, while a chain with two or three double bonds (e.g.,

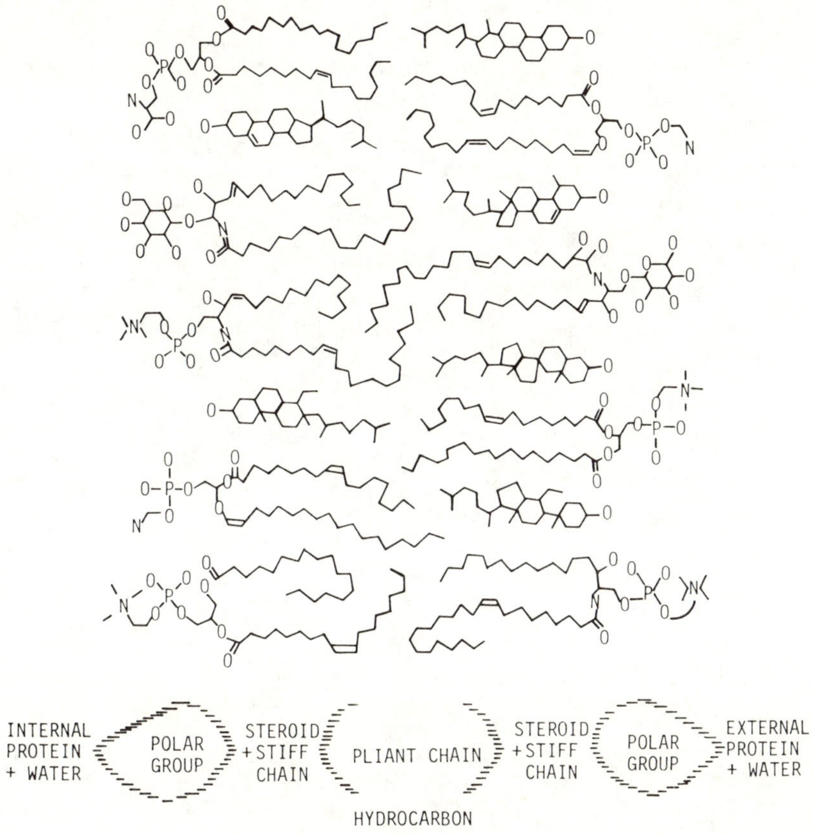

FIGURE 4. Schematic structure of a membrane.

18:2 or 18:3) cannot. This may be the explanation why the interaction of cholesterol with phospholipids decreases as the degree of unsaturation increases and why cholesterol condenses monolayers of lecithin-di-oleyl (PC-di 18:1) but not lecithin-di-linoleyl (PC-di 18:2). The disposition of cholesterol will therefore depend on the unsaturation of the phospholipid. For instance one would expect more cholesterol in the vicinity of sphingomyelin than near more highly unsaturated lecithin. One might also expect clustering of cholesterol because of its strong tendency for self-association.[28]

C. Asymmetry

The membrane in the fluid-mosaic model appears structurally uniform in its plane, with considerable freedom for lateral motion, but is highly ordered if viewed in a direction perpendicular to its plane. This structural anisotropy may determine many of the functional properties.

1. Transverse

The distribution of the individual membrane components has been found to be asymmetric in relation to the inner and outer leaflets of the lipid bilayer. This has been assumed for some time on the basis of the asymmetric functions of a membrane since the two faces of the membrane face different tasks. It has now become clear that the structural asymmetry is extensive and involves all major components of the membrane.[29] The evidence has been obtained primarily for the red cell. However, recent results with enveloped animal viruses, mitochondria, endoplasmic reticulum, platelets,

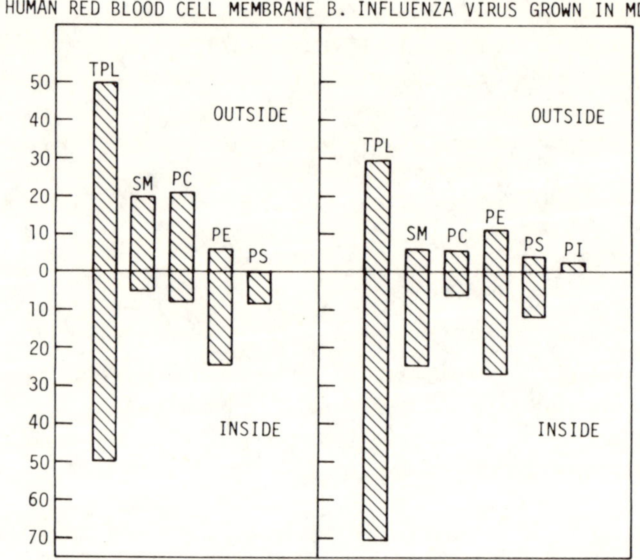

FIGURE 5. Transmembrane asymmetry of phospholipids. Asymmetrical distribution of phospholipids in membranes of human red blood cells and influenza virus grown in MDBK cells, expressed as mol percent. Abbreviations: TPL, total phospholipid; PC, phosphatidylcholine; SM, sphingomyelin; PE, phosphatidylethanolamine; PS, phosphatidylserine; and PI, phosphatidylinositol. (From Rothman, J. and Lenard, J., *Science*, 195, 743, 1977. With permission.)

sarcoplasmic reticulum, lymphocyte plasma membrane, intestinal brush border, and bacterial membranes indicate that similar structural principles may apply to most biological membranes.[30] Carbohydrates have been found exclusively on the red cell outer surface;[31] consequently, those lipids and proteins containing carbohydrates must likewise be on that side.

Proteins of the red cell have been found that are present only on the outer surface, only on the inner surface, or spanning the membrane with different polypeptides on the two membrane surfaces (Reference 5, Volume 1, Chapter 10). Similarly, the two major Proteins of myelin have been found to be located asymmetrically and to interact with different lipids.[30] This asymmetry of proteins as well as of carbohydrates is absolute. No portion of a polypeptide chain (or of a carbohydrate) is present on both halves of the bilayer.

The evidence for the asymmetric distribution of phospholipids is by now very convincing for RBC, some virions, gram-positive bacilli, and for myelin. For all of them it has been shown by several independent methods that the more cationic phospholipids, lecithin and sphingomyelin, are preferentially exposed on the outer surface, while phosphatidylethanolamine and phosphatidylserine with ionizable primary amino groups are primarily on the inner surface (Figure 5).[32,33] Some recent studies suggest caution in the interpretation of results when phospholipases are used for the elucidation of the precise structural details of the phospholipid bilayer.[34]

Much less is known about the location of cholesterol. For RBC it has been concluded on the basis of exchange reactions that the outer leaflet is richer in cholesterol than the inner one.[35] Similarly for myelin it has been shown on the basis of X-ray diffraction data that the ratio of cholesterol/polar phospholipid is 1:1 at the outside but 3:7 at the inside of the membrane.[36] Electron micrographs of freeze-etched, specially prepared RBC also indicate a larger proportion of cholesterol in the outer than the inner leaflet.[37] Such an asymmetry would be expected because of the interactions of cholesterol with the asymmetrically distributed phospholipids and proteins.

On the other hand, a study using OsO_4-esters of cholesterol to localize cholesterol in rat RBC indicates that it is dispersed in clusters and distributed throughout the thickness of the membrane,[38] and kinetic studies of ^{14}C-cholesterol transport from phosphatidylcholine vesicles to RBCs[39] suggest that cholesterol is present in two pools of comparable size, probably reflecting cholesterol in the inner and outer leaflets. Similarly, evidence has been presented that 50 to 66% of the cholesterol in some mycoplasma species is located in the outer half of the membrane[40] and that cholesterol in influenza virus membranes distributes only slowly between the inner and outer leaflets.[41]

2. Lateral

There is also evidence for asymmetry in the lateral distribution of components within the plane of the membrane. Most studies refer to heterogeneity of distribution of proteins. Examples are clustering of receptor sites for lectins and concanavalin A,[42] and capping of antigens on lymphoid cells and on fibroblasts[43] (for review see Reference 44).

Examples for lateral asymmetry of lipids as distinguished from lateral mobility in biological membranes are sparse. Murphy's study of the distribution of cholesterol in RBC[45] showing a higher concentration around the ''dimple'' must be considered equivocal because the experimental data permit several different interpretations. The possibility of its occurrence is however supported by experiments in model systems, showing preferential interactions of cholesterol with specific phospholipids. In mixtures, this leads to the nonrandom distribution of cholesterol under conditions where there occurs a phase separation of the phospholipids. This means that under these conditions there is the formation of clusters of phospholipid-cholesterol complexes.[25,47]

An attractive hypothesis for the formation of echinocytes in cholesterol-loaded RBC (Figure 6)[48] is an asymmetric disposition of cholesterol. This could be a lateral or a transverse asymmetry. A lateral asymmetry would form cholesterol-enriched and -depleted domains that could permit formation of the spurs by local weakening of the orderly organization of the bilayer or local inhomogeneities of surface tension properties. The observation that reversible spurring by the action of anionic or noncharged amphiphilic substances occurs at the same place on the membrane[49] would support this hypothesis. On the other hand, it has been shown that echinocytes are formed whenever the surface area of the outer leaflet of the membrane is increased in relation to that of the inner leaflet.[50] By that token, an asymmetric addition of cholesterol to the outer leaflet would account for the shape change in response to cholesterol-loading.

V. EFFECTS OF CHOLESTEROL IN MEMBRANES

The major function of cholesterol in membranes is now thought to be the control it exerts on the interactions of its components. It affects the mobility of the hydrocarbon chains of the phospholipids and to some degree the spacing of the polar head groups,[24] the lipid-protein interactions, and possibly even protein-protein interactions (see enzymes). In short, cholesterol affects the ''fluidity'' or ''microviscosity'' of membranes. Fluidity is of course also affected by the kind of fatty acid present and therefore by the kind of phospholipid since phospholipid classes tend to be characterized by the degree of unsaturation of their hydrocarbon chains.

A. Molecular Surface Area

Early observations leading to the hypothesis that cholesterol affects membrane fluidity were those concerning the surface area of monomolecular films of lipids. Choles-

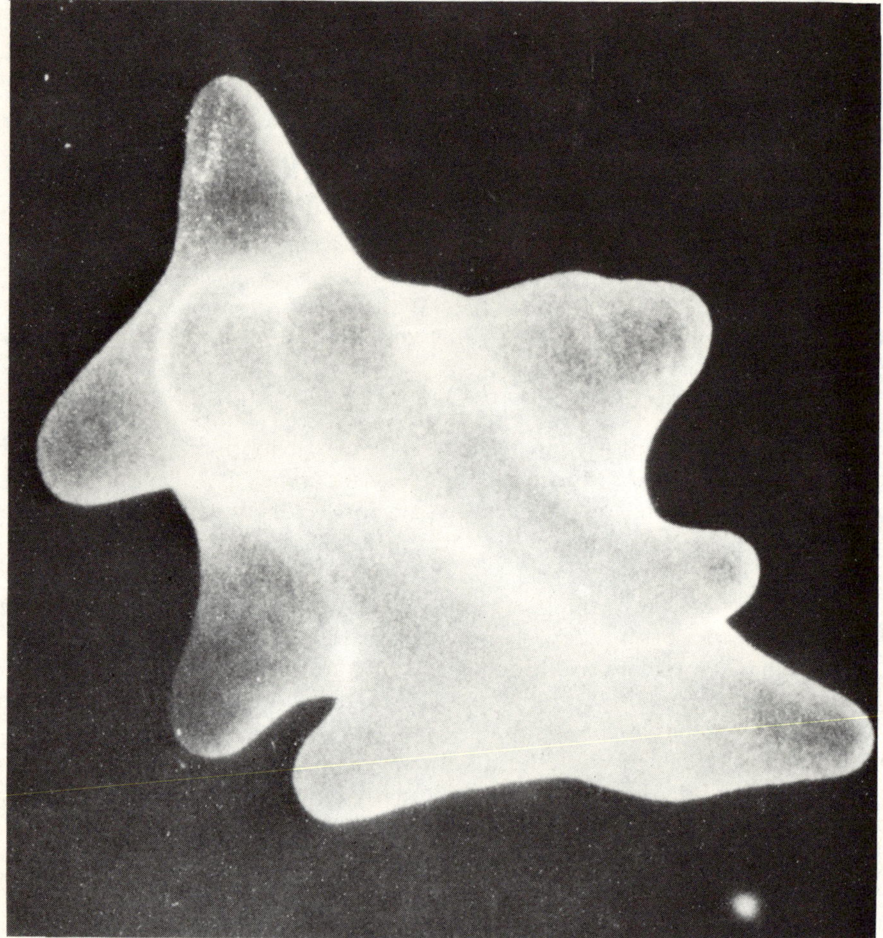

FIGURE 6. Cholesterol-loaded red cells from guinea pigs fed cholesterol.
A. X6000

terol forms a liquid, condensed film with very little compressibility.[51] The molecular area of phospholipids in films depends primarily on the fatty acid constituents although the polar head groups do have an effect. Long-chain saturated fatty acids produce the most condensed films (the smallest area). Shorter-chain fatty acids and the introduction of double bonds increase the area per molecule. The addition of cholesterol to phospholipid monolayers alters their molcular area (at a given pressure) (Figure 7), that is, in a mixed monomolecular film containing phospholipid and cholesterol the average area per molecule is usually smaller than the sum of the areas of the components.

B. Phase Changes, Fluidity

Lipid bilayers of artificial vesicles or biological membranes undergo reversible transitions from a more ordered, quasi-crystalline to a disordered, liquid crystalline state at a characteristic critical temperature, T_c (Figure 8).[52] Such phase transitions are accompanied by the release or consumption of energy in the exothermic reactions of "crystallization" or "melting" respectively. Study of model systems by differential scanning calorimetry has shown that the addition of cholesterol to phospholipid decreases the amount of energy required for the crystalline → liquid crystalline phase

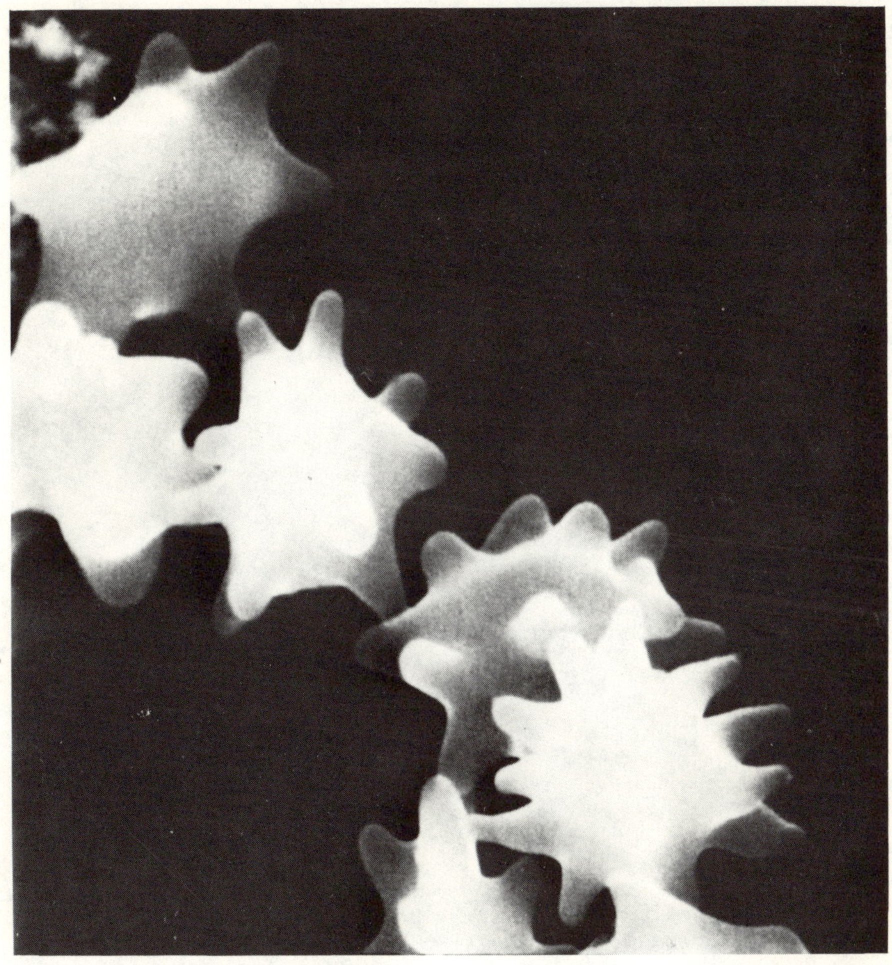

B. X20,000.

and therefore to lower the transition temperature.[53] This has been interpreted to indicate that the effects of cholesterol on the molecular area of phospholipids and on their transition temperatures are due to a decrease of the strength of the hydrophobic bonds between the phospholipid tails by the intercalation of cholesterol. That is, in the presence of cholesterol, these hydrocarbon chains are more mobile, therefore using more space and are more disordered, therefore more "fluid." On the other hand, cholesterol will increase the packing of more unsaturated fatty acid chains and thus will increase the temperature for the liquid → crystalline transition and will increase the amount of heat released. More generally, cholesterol exerts a dual effect decreasing the fluidity of the hydrocarbon chains above their transition temperature (where they are fluid) and increasing their fluidity below it (where they are in the gel state) (Figure 9) (Reference 5, Volume 2, Chapter 1). The largest increase in rigidity has been found to be in the middle of the fatty acid chain.[54] This is one of the observations suggesting the position of cholesterol as shown in Figure 4. At high cholesterol concentrations, the state of fluidity is intermediate between the more rigid gel phase and the less rigid liquid-crystalline phase. The thermal transition is abolished at cholesterol/phospholipid ratios above 1:1 or 1:2, depending on the author.[55,56] In addition, such cholesterol-phospholipid mixtures are dispersible in water over a wider range of temperature than the individual components.[53]

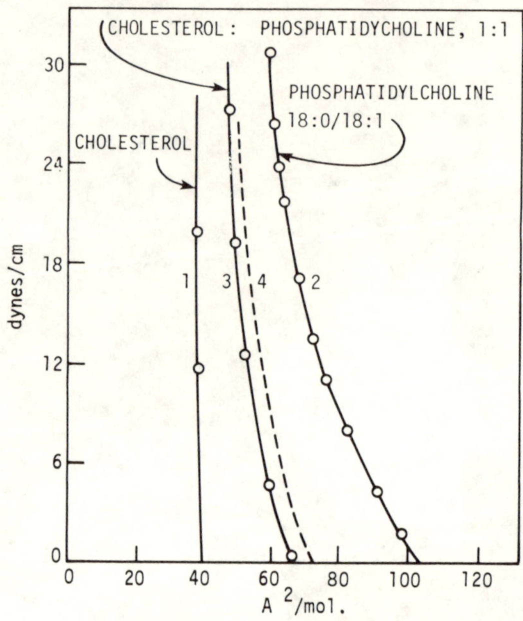

FIGURE 7. Condensing effect of cholesterol on lipid monolayers. Pressure vs. area characteristics of monolayers of cholesterol, stearoyloleoylphosphatidylcholine and an equimolar mixture of the two lipids. 1, cholesterol; 2, stearoyloleoylphosphatidylcholine; 3, equimolar mixture of cholesterol and stearoyloleoylphosphatidylcholine; 4, proportionate average of the curves for the two pure lipids. It shows a) that cholesterol has very little compressibility, e.g. the area remains constant with increasing pressure and b) that for the same pressure the area of a mixed film is smaller than for the pure phospholipid (compare 2 and 3) and smaller than the proportionate average of 2 pure lipids. (From Demel, R. A. and de Kruyff, B., *Biochim. Biophys. Acta*, 457, 109, 1976. With permission.)

These results have been obtained by several methods and both in model systems as well as in biological membranes. For instance, changes of microviscosity can be observed directly by fluorescence polarization[57] and phase changes can be visualized by freeze-fracture electron microscopy.[58] Electronspin resonance (ESR), proton nuclear magnetic resonance (^{1}H-NMR) and ^{13}C-NMR studies of oriented multilayers, liposomes, and vesicles of phospholipids have shown that the degree of order was increased by the addition of cholesterol to a system like egg lecithin that is in the liquid-crystalline state at room temperature. (For a review of methods see Reference 59.) A similar condensing effect of cholesterol has recently been observed in complexes of phospholipid and protein in the case of dimyristoyl-lecithin (PC-di 14:0) and apolipoprotein A-I.[60] Conversely, the presence of cholesterol increased spin probe separations and mobility of dipalmitoyl-lecithin (PC-di 16:0) systems that are in the gel state at room temperature (below T_c) (see review, Reference 1).

Similar results have been obtained in biological membranes, for instance by ESR studies in strains of *M. mycoides* high or low in cholesterol and in cholesterol-loaded RBC from guinea pigs.[59,61,62] A good correlation of microviscosity as measured by fluorescence polarization and cholesterol/phospholipid ratio has been reported for hu-

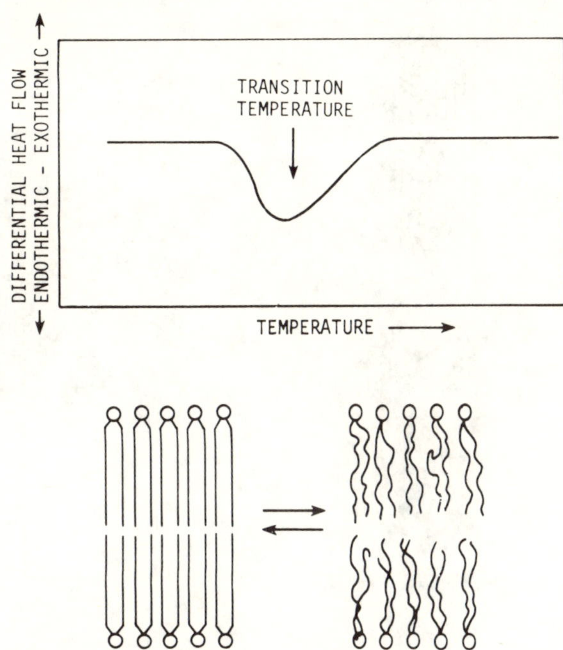

FIGURE 8. Thermotropic transitions of amphipathic lipids. The diagram shows an idealized calorimeter scan of amphipathic lipids indicating the endothermic transition from the crystalline to the liquid crystalline phase. The lower scheme shows the state of the lipids at temperatures lower (left) and higher (right) than the critical transition temperature. (From Lenaz, G., *Acta Vitam. Enzymol. (Milano)*, 27, 62, 1973. With permission.)

man red cell membranes (Figure 10).[63] Evidence has been accumulating that a structure transition occurs in a lipid bilayer if the ratio of cholesterol to phospholipid exceeds about 0.33 mol fraction of cholesterol. The studies have used X-ray diffraction,[64] calorimetry,[65] NMR,[66] fluorescence polarization,[59] and complement-mediated attack on haptens,[67] and the results have been interpreted to indicate that at the higher ratios of cholesterol/phospholipid there may be domains specifically enriched or depleted of cholesterol.

The fluidity of membranes controls the stability, stiffness, deformability, and even shape of cells and a number of their functional properties such as permeability to metabolites and nutrients, ion transport, endocytosis, and receptor availability that can in turn affect immunological responses, cell-cell recognition and cell differentiation and the activity of membrane-associated enzymes.

1. Permeability

The permeability of liposomes to glucose was greatly decreased when cholesterol was added to phospholipids, such as palmityl-oleyl-lecithin (PC-16:0, 18:1), that interact with cholesterol but was not affected in the case of dilinoleyl-lecithin (PC-di 18:2). Similar results were found for the permeability to glycerol and erythritol and for the activation energy of diffusion for Na^+, K^+, and Cl^- in vesicles from beef brain phosphatidylserine (PS).[1,68] In general, below the phase transition of a particular lecithin, the presence of cholesterol in liposomes enhances solute transfer, whereas the opposite effect is obtained above the phase transition temperature.[55,68]

The permeability of biological membranes is affected by cholesterol similar to that

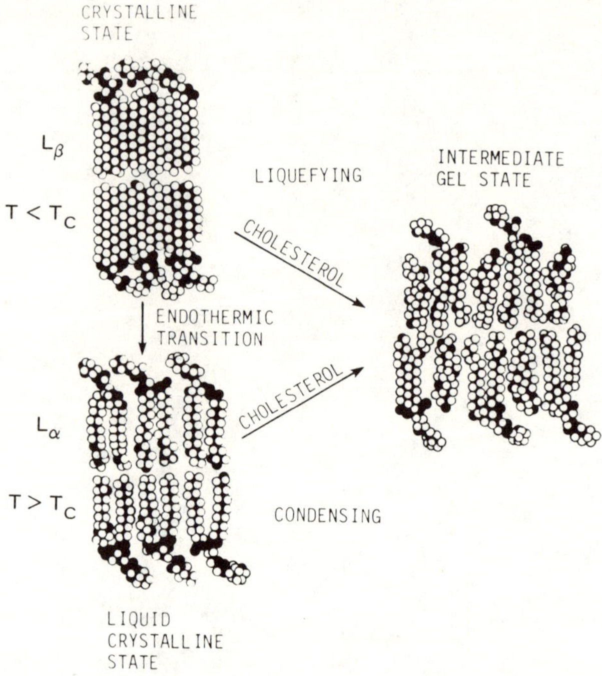

FIGURE 9. Representation by molecular models of the liquefying and condensing effect of cholesterol. (From Demel, R. A. and deKruyff, B., Biochim. Biophys. Acta, 457, 109, 1976. With permission.)

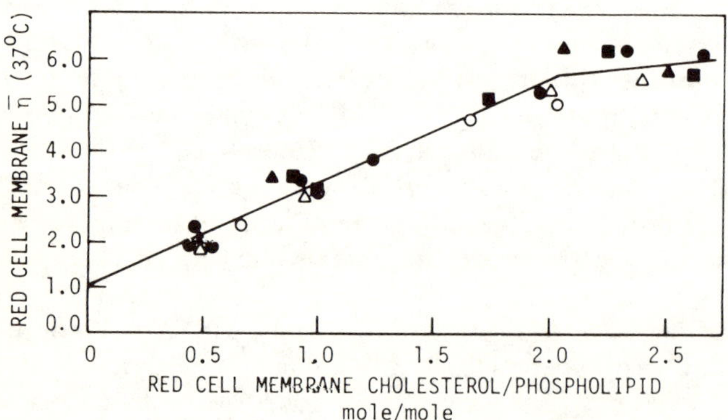

FIGURE 10. Effect of cholesterol content on membrane viscosity. Effect of the cholesterol:phospholipid mol ratio of red cell membranes on effective membrane viscosity ($\bar{\eta}$) at 37°C. Red cells were incubated with dispersions of cholesterol and various phospholipids. (o) egg lecithin; (•) L-dipalmitoyllecithin; (▲) DL-dipalmitoyllecithin; (■) L-dimyristolylecithin, and (△) bovine brain sphingomyelin. (From Cooper, R., Leslie, M., Fischkoff, S., Shintzky, M., and Shattil, S., *Biochemistry,* 17, 327, 1978. With permission.)

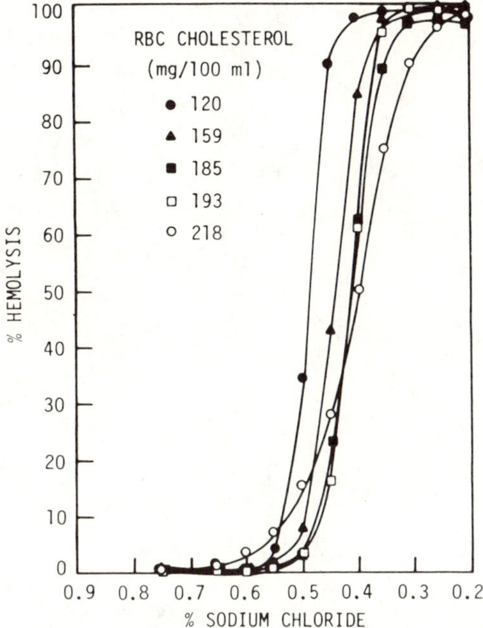

FIGURE 11. Effect of cholesterol content on osmotic fragility of red cells. Red cells of guinea pigs were loaded with cholesterol by feeding them a cholesterol-containing diet for varying periods of time. The figure shows that with increasing cholesterol content the cells withstand increasing hypotonicity. (From Aswad, C. and Ostwald, R., *J. Clin. Invest.*, 55, 115, 1975. With permission.)

of these model systems. In *Acholeplasma laidlawii,* as well as in guinea pig RBC, increased proportions of cholesterol/phospholipid cause a decrease of their permeability of Na^+ ion and to some nonelectrolytes.[11,69] Conversely, partial removal of cholesterol from human RBC increased glycerol permeability[13] and diffusion of anionic substances.[70]

Water permeability of both liposomes and biological membranes is also controlled in part by their fluidity and therefore affected by the presence of cholesterol.

2. Stability, Stiffness

The effects of cholesterol on membrane fluidity as expressed in stability, stiffness, and deformability have been most extensively investigated in RBC. These membranes are not only obtainable easily and in large amounts but are also uncontaminated with intracellular membranes such as mitochondria or microsomes. Cholesterol-loaded RBC have an increased resistance to osmotic lysis (Figure 11),[72,73] to shear stress, and to filterability, indicating an increased internal viscosity. Cholesterol-depleted RBC show changes in the opposite direction. Intestinal microvillus membranes, which are more rigid than most others, have been reported to have a high cholesterol/phospholipid ratio,[74] indicating again that cholesterol affects this parameter.

The stability of lysosomes, the intracellular structures containing catabolic enzymes, is greatly increased by cholesterol. The importance of membrane cholesterol in this connection has been established by the observation that incubation of rat liver lysosomes in the presence of digitonin or polyene antibiotics labilizes their membranes as shown by leakage of acid phosphatase. This effect is presumably due to the complexing of cholesterol by these agents (Reference 5, Volume 2, Chapter 5; 71).

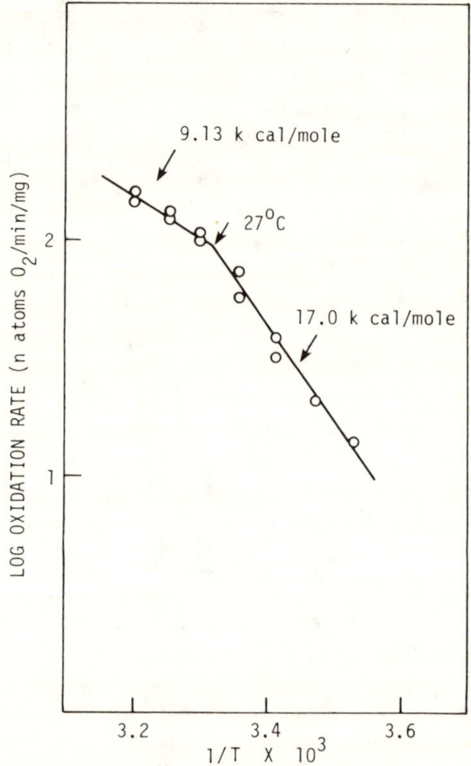

FIGURE 12. Arrhenius plot of succinoxidase activity in beef heart mitochondria. (From Lenaz, G. *Acta Vitam. Enzymd. (Milano)*, 27, 62, 1973. With permission.)

3. Enzyme Activities

The fluidity of membranes (and therefore cholesterol) also contributes to the control of the function of their protein components. About 30 enzymes have been shown to be lipid-dependent as judged by their inactivation following lipid removal and reactivation by relipidation.[2,53,75] This lipid requirement however is frequently nonspecific, and in many cases membrane lipids can even be replaced by detergents for the reactivation of delipidized enzymes.[23]

Much of the transport of materials across membranes involves either facilitated or active transport. Two important transport systems are those for Na and K ions, by the Na^+K^+ATPases, the other for Ca^{++} by the Ca^+ATPase. Both of these enzyme systems have been shown to require phospholipids for activity.[2] The rate of the reaction depends on the fluidity of the surrounding lipids. In the case of lamb kidney Na^+K^+ATPase, the rate was found to be one third when the lipids were below their transition temperature compared to the reaction at a temperature above their transition temperature.[76] The change in rates in many but not all instances occurs abruptly, e.g., there is a discontinuity in the Arrhenius plot, and occurs at the same temperature as the gel → liquid transition (Figure 12).[52] This indicates that the transition is characteristic for the lipids and not for the protein. Similar results have been obtained for bacterial membranes as well as for some mitochondrial enzymes.[77]

An involvement of cholesterol in the activity of membrane enzymes, presumably by its effects on membrane fluidity, has also been suggested by the results of studies showing a decrease of adenylate cyclase and Na^+ K^+ ATPase activities in human fibroblasts and rabbit kidney cells enriched with cholesterol.[16,17] A very recent study reported that both the release of arachidonic acid from phospholipids and the production of thromboxane A_2 was greater in cholesterol-enriched compared to cholesterol-depleted platelets.[80] This implies an effect of membrane cholesterol on the activities of phospholipase A_2 and thromboxane synthetase.

The fluidity of its surroundings could affect enzyme activity by several mechanisms. The microviscosity will control the diffusion or rotation of both the enzyme molecules and of the substrate. This would apply particularly strongly to the latter if it is a hydrophobic substrate located in the lipid domain. The conformation of the enzyme and therefore its catalytic activity, stability, and sensitivity to inhibitors or activators may be affected by the physical state of the activating lipid (Reference 5, Volume 2, Chapter 1; 17). This is suggested for instance by experiments showing that the cholesterol content of the diet affects the allosteric inhibition by fluoride of the Na^+K^+ATPase of rat RBC.[78] The influence of fatty acyl chain fluidity on enzyme function has been termed viscotropic regulation.[79] It is important to remember that the term fluidity is rather loosely defined and its magnitude is expressed by a variety of parameters that may or may not measure the same properties: spectral order parameters, relaxation times, partition coefficients of probe molecules, diffusion coefficients, critical temperatures, etc.[81]

4. Immunological Response

Cholesterol content and fluidity of a membrane affect other functions of the membrane. One of the most intriguing ones is the effect of fluidity on immunological behavior. Liposomes of PC-di 16:0 in the presence of small amounts of cardiolipin as the hapten were found to bind increasing amounts of complement with increasing concentration of cholesterol above 33 mol %.[67] Analogous studies have reported changes of binding of antibodies to lipid hapten-sensitized liposomal membranes as a function of host lipid composition.[82] These results were interpreted to be caused by the increasing inhibition of the lateral motion of the hapten. The fact that such translational diffusion exists had been shown previously by attaching fluorescent antibody to the antigen in tissue culture cells.[42] This interpretation is in accord with other evidence that the fluidity is governed by the lipid composition and that it controls to a major degree the lateral and rotational mobility of receptor sites.[83] There are however alternative explanations for an altered immune response caused by changes in cholesterol/phospholipid ratios. It may be caused by exposing cryptic antigenic sites[84] or by major structural reorganization.[82] Still another mechanism is suggested by the observation that cholesterol-loaded lymphocytes had a decreased degree of responsiveness as measured by binding of concanavalin A[85] and may therefore be expected to have altered responses to other stimuli.

5. Cell Division

Another interesting wrinkle in the cholesterol story is indirect evidence that there may be a requirement by cells for an increment in the amount of cholesterol during cell division. DNA synthesis and cell division is suppressed in several systems when the cells are grown in cholesterol-free media and treated with inhibitors of cholesterol synthesis.[86] Whether the requirement for cholesterol in the formation of new membrane is the sole reason for this phenomenon is not known. Nor is it clear how DNA synthesis may be regulated by some function of the plasma membrane although several authors have speculated on the subject (for review, see Reference 87). One attractive hypothesis is the involvement of cyclic AMP that is thought to contribute to the control of cell growth and division because there is evidence that cholesterol is involved in the activation of adenyl cyclase by hormones.[88]

VI. SUMMARY

Present evidence indicates that all biological membranes share the same structural principle visualized as a sandwich formed by phospholipids and usually cholesterol, interrupted by proteins on either side or spanning the entire bilayer. There is a certain degree of asymmetry in the distribution of the major components both laterally, in the plane of the membrane, and transversely, in the two leaflets of the bilayer. This structure is dictated by the hydrophobic and hydrophilic forces acting between and among the lipid and protein components. The specific function of cholesterol appears to be the control it exerts over the fluidity (or microviscosity) of the membrane. The stiffness (deformability) of cell membranes, the stability of plasma and intracellular membranes, the permeability to and transport of ions as well as nonionic compounds, the activity of a number of membrane enzymes, and a number of surface phenomena such as immunological responses and cell-cell interactions, all depend to some degree on the appropriate fluidity of the membrane and so on the proper amount of cholesterol.

ACKNOWLEDGMENT

I am grateful to Dr. Joan Tinoco for reading the manuscript and for helpful suggestions for its improvement.

REFERENCES

1. **Demel, R. A. and de Kruyff, B.,** The function of sterols in membranes, *Biochim. Biophys. Acta,* 457, 109, 1976.
2. **Masoro, E. J.,** Lipids and lipid metabolism, *Ann. Rev. Physiol.,* 39, 301, 1977.
3. **Stoeckenius, W. and Engelman, D.,** Current models for the structure of biological membranes, *J. Cell Biol.,* 42, 613, 1969.
4. **Philipps, C.,** The physical state of phospholipids and cholesterol in monolayers, bilayers, and membranes, *Prog. Surf. Membrane Sci.,* 5, 139, 1972.
5. **Jamieson, G. and Robinson, D., Eds.,** *Mammalian Cell Membranes,* Vols. 1, 2 (1976); Vols. 3, 4, 5, Butterworths, London, 1977.
6. **Snyder, F., Ed.,** *Lipid Metabolism in Mammals,* Plenum Press, New York, 1977.
7. **Steck, T. and Fox, C.,** Membrane proteins, in *Membrane Molecular Biology,* Fox, C. and Keith, A., Eds., Sinauer Associates, Stamford, Connecticut, 1972, 27.
8. **Rouser, G., Nelson, G., and Fleischer, S.,** Lipid composition of animal cell membranes, organelles, and organs, in *Biological Membranes,* Chapman, D., Ed., Academic Press, New York, 1968, 5.
9. **Ansell, G., Hawthorne, J., and Dawson, R.,** Form and function of phospholipids, *Biochim. Biophys. Acta Library,* Vol. 3, Elsevier, Amsterdam, 1973.
10. **Nelson, G.,** Lipid composition and metabolism of erythrocytes, in *Blood Lipids and Lipoproteins,* Nelson, G., Ed., Wiley-Interscience, New York, 1972, chap. 7.
11. **de Kruyff, B., de Greef, W., van Eyke, R., Demel, R., and van Deenen, L.,** The effect of different fatty acid and sterol composition on the effect of the erythritol flux through the cell membrane of *Acholeplasma laidlawii, Biochim. Biophys. Acta,* 298, 479, 1973.
12. **Cobon, G. and Haslam, J.,** The effect of altered membrane sterol composition on the temperature dependence of yeast mitochondrial ATP-ase, *Biochem. Biophys. Res. Commun.,* 52, 320, 1973.
13. **Bruckdorfer, K., Demel, R., de Gier, J., and van Deenen, L.,** The effect of partial replacements of membrane cholesterol by other steroids on the osmotic fragility and glycerol permeability of erythrocytes, *Biochim. Biophys. Acta,* 183, 334, 1969.
14. **Sardet, C., Hansma, H., and Ostwald, R.,** Effects of plasma lipoproteins from control and cholesterol-fed guinea pigs on red cell morphology and cholesterol content: An in vitro study, *J. Lipid Res.,* 13, 705, 1972.

15. **Cooper, R., Arner, E., Wiley, J., and Shattil, S.,** Modification of red cell membrane structure by cholesterol-rich lipid dispersions, *J. Clin. Invest.*, 55, 115, 1975.
16. **Klein, I., Moore, L., and Pastan, I.,** Effect of liposomes containing cholesterol on adenylate cyclase activity of cultured mammalian fibroblasts, *Biochim. Biophys. Acta*, 506, 42, 1978.
17. **Kimelberg, H.,** Alterations in phospholipid-dependent (Na^+ + K^+)-ATPase activity due to lipid fluidity. Effects of cholesterol and Mg^{2+}, *Biochim. Biophys. Acta*, 413, 143, 1975.
18. **Graham, J. and Green, C.,** The properties of mitochondria enriched in vitro with cholesterol, *Eur. J. Biochem.*, 12, 58, 1970.
19. **Ostwald, R. and Shannon, A.,** Composition of tissue lipids and anemia of guinea pigs in response to dietary cholesterol, *Biochem. J.*, 91, 146, 1964.
20. **Neerhout, R.,** Abnormalities of erythrocyte stromal lipids in hepatic disease, *J. Lab. Clin. Med.*, 71, 438, 1968.
21. **Tanford, C.,** Thermodynamics of micelle formation: Prediction of micelle size and size distribution, *Proc. Nat. Acad. Sci. U.S.A.*, 71, 1811, 1974.
22. **Singer, S.,** The molecular organization of biological membranes, in *Structure and Function of Biological Membranes*, Rothfield, L., Ed., Academic Press, New York, 1971, 145.
23. **Singer, S. and Nicolson, G.,** The fluid mosaic model of the structure of cell membranes, *Science*, 175, 720, 1972.
24. **Yeagle, P., Hutton, W., Huang, C-H., and Martin, R.,** Phospholipid headgroup conformations: Intermolecular interactions and cholesterol effects, *Biochemistry*, 16, 4344, 1977.
25. **Darke, A., Finer, E., Flook, A., and Philipps, M.,** Complex and cluster formation in mixed lecithin cholesterol bilayers. Cooperativity of motion in lipid systems, *FEBS Lett.*, 18, 326, 1971.
26. **Huang, C-H.,** A structural model for the cholesterol-phosphatidylcholine complexes in bilayer membranes, *Lipids*, 12, 348, 1977.
27. **London, Y., Demel, R., Geurts van Kessel, W., Zahler, P., and van Deenen, L.,** The interaction of the Folch-Lees protein with lipids at the air water interface, *Biochim. Biophys. Acta*, 332, 69, 1974.
28. **Haberlund, M. and Reynolds, J.,** Self-association of cholesterol in aqueous solution, *Proc. Nat. Acad. Sci. U.S.A.*, 70, 2313, 1973.
29. **Rothman, J. and Lenard, J.,** Membrane asymmetry, *Science*, 195, 743, 1977.
30. **Demel, R., London, Y., Geurts van Kessel, W., Vossenberg, F., and van Deenen, L.,** The specific interaction of myelin basic protein with lipids at the air-water interface, *Biochim. Biophys. Acta*, 311, 507, 1973.
31. **Nicolson, G. and Singer, S.,** Ferritin-conjugated plant agglutinins as specific saccharide stains for electron microscopy: Application to saccharides bound to cell membranes, *Proc. Nat. Acad. Sci. U.S.A.*, 68, 942, 1971.
32. **Bretscher, M.,** Membrane structure: Some general principles, *Science*, 181, 622, 1973.
33. **Zwaal, R., Roelofson, B., and Colley, C.,** Localization of red cell membrane constituents, *Biochim. Biophys. Acta*, 300, 159, 1973.
34. **Adamich, M. and Dennis, E.,** Exploring the action and specificity of cobra venom phospholipase A_2 toward human RBC, ghost membranes and lipid mixtures, *J. Biol. Chem.*, 253, 5121, 1978.
35. **Murphy, J.,** Erythrocyte metabolism. IV. Equilibration of cholesterol-4-^{14}C between erythrocytes and variously treated sera, *J. Lab. Clin. Med.*, 60, 571, 1962.
36. **Caspar, D. and Kirschner, D.,** Myelin membrane structure at 10 A resolution, *Nat. N. Biol.*, 231, 46, 1971.
37. **Fisher, K.,** Analysis of membrane halves: Cholesterol, *Proc. Nat. Acad. Sci. U.S.A.*, 73, 173, 1976.
38. **Higgins, J., Florendo, N., and Barnett, R.,** Localization of cholesterol in membranes of erythrocyte ghosts, *J. Ulstrastruc. Res.*, 42, 66, 1973.
39. **Bloj, B. and Zilversmit, D.,** Transposition and distribution of cholesterol in rat erythrocytes, *Proc. Soc. Exp. Biol. Med.*, 156, 539, 1977.
40. **Bittman, R. and Rottem, S.,** Distribution of cholesterol between the outer and inner halves of the lipid bilayer of mycoplasma cell membranes, *Biochem. Biophys. Res. Commun.*, 71, 318, 1976.
41. **Lenard, J. and Rothman, J.,** Transbilayer distribution and movement of cholesterol and phospholipid in the membrane of influenza virus, *Proc. Nat. Acad. Sci. U.S.A.*, 73, 391, 1976.
42. **Frye, L. and Edidin, M.,** The rapid intermixing of cell surface antigens after formation of mouse-human heterokaryons, *J. Cell Sci.*, 7, 319, 1970.
43. **Taylor, R., Duffus, W., Raff, M., and de Petris, S.,** Redistribution and pinocytosis of lymphocyte surface immunoglobulin molecules induced by anti-immunoglobulin antibody, *Nat. N. Biol.*, 233, 225, 1971.
44. **Nicolson, G.,** Transmembrane control of the receptors on normal and tumor cells. 1. Cytoplasmic influence over cell surface components, *Biochim. Biophys. Acta.*, 457, 57, 1976.
45. **Murphy, J.,** Erythrocyte metabolism. IV. Cell shape and the location of cholesterol in the erythrocyte membrane, *J. Lab. Clin. Med.*, 65, 756, 1965.

46. **de Kruyff, B., van Dijck, P., Demel, R., Schnijff, A., Brants, F., and van Deenen, L.,** Nonrandom distribution of cholesterol in phosphatidylcholine bylayers, *Biochim. Biophys. Acta,* 356, 1, 1974.
47. **Shimshick, E. and McConnell, H.,** Lateral phase separation in binary mixtures of cholesterol and phospholipids, *Biochem. Biophys. Res. Commun.,* 53, 446, 1973.
48. **McBride, J. and Jacob, H.,** Abnormal kinetics of red cell membrane cholesterol in acanthocytes: Studies in genetic and experimental abetalipoproteinaemia and in spur cell anemia, *Brit. J. Haematol.,* 18, 383, 1970.
49. **Bessis, M. and Prenant, M.,** Topography of the appearance of spicules in crenated erythrocytes, *Nouv. Rev. Franc. d'Hemat.,* 12, 351, 1972.
50. **Sheetz, M. and Singer, S.,** Biological membranes as bilayer couples. A molecular mechanism of drug-erythrocyte interactions, *Proc. Nat. Acad. Sci. U.S.A.,* 71, 4457, 1974.
51. **Pethica, B.,** The thermodynamics of monolayer penetration at constant area, *Trans. Faraday Soc.,* 51, 1402, 1955.
52. **Lenaz, G.,** The role of lipids in the regulation of membrane-associated activities, *Acta Vitam. Enzymol. (Milano),* 27, 62, 1973.
53. **Ladbrooke, B., Williams, R., and Chapman, D.** Studies of lecithin-cholesterol-water interactions by differential scanning calorimetry and x-ray diffraction, *Biochim. Biophys. Acta,* 150, 333, 1968.
54. **Godici, P. and Landsberger, F.,** ^{13}C-nuclear magnetic resonance study of the dynamic structure of lecithin-cholesterol membranes and the position of steric acid spin labels, *Biochemistry,* 14, 3927, 1975.
55. **Chapman, D.,** Some recent studies of lipids, lipid-cholesterol, and membrane systems, in *Biological Membranes,* Vol. 2, Chapman, D. and Wallach, D., Eds., Academic Press, New York, 1973, Chap. 2.
56. **Hinz, H. and Sturtevant, J.,** Calorimetric investigation of the influence of cholesterol on transition properties of bilayers formed from synthetic L-α-lecithins in aqueous suspensions, *J. Biol. Chem.,* 247, 3697, 1972.
57. **Shinitzky, M. and Inbar, M.,** Microviscosity parameters and protein mobility in biological membranes, *Biochim. Biophys. Acta,* 433, 133, 1976.
58. **Verkley, A., Ververgaert, P., van Deenen, L., and Elbers, P.,** Phase transitions of phospholipid bilayers and membranes of *Acholeplasma laidlawii B* visualized by freeze fracturing electron microscopy, *Biochim. Biophys. Acta,* 288, 326, 1972.
59. **Andersen, H.,** Probes of membrane structure, *Ann. Rev. Biochem.,* 47, 359, 1978.
60. **Jonas, A. and Krajnovich, D.,** Effect of cholesterol on the formation of micellar complexes between bovine A-1 apoliproprotein and L-α-dimyristoyl-phosphatidylcholine, *J. Biol. Chem.,* 253, 5758, 1978.
61. **Rottem, S., Cirillo, V., de Kruyff, B., Shinitzky, M., and Razin, S.,** Cholesterol in mycoplasma membranes, *Biochim. Biophys. Acta,* 323, 509, 1973.
62. **Kroes, J., Ostwald, R., and Keith, A.,** Erythrocyte membranes. Compression of lipid phases by increased cholesterol content, *Biochim. Biophys. Acta,* 274, 71, 1972.
63. **Cooper, R., Leslie, M., Fischkoff, S., Shinitzky, M., and Shattil, S.,** Factors influencing the lipid composition and fluidity of red cell membranes in vitro: Production of red cells possessing more than two cholesterols per phospholipid, *Biochemistry,* 17, 327, 1978.
64. **Engleman, D. and Rothman, J.,** The planar organization of lecithin-cholesterol bilayers, *J. Biol. Chem.,* 247, 3694, 1972.
65. **Hinz, H. and Sturtevant, J.,** Calormetric investigation of the influence of cholesterol on the transition properties of bilayers formed from synthetic L-α-lecithins in aqueous suspensions, *J. Biol. Chem.,* 247, 3697, 1972.
66. **Taylor, R., Huang, C-H., Broccoli, A., and Leake, L.,** Nuclear magnetic resonance studies on amphiphile hydration, *Arch. Biochem. Biophys.,* 183, 83, 1977.
67. **Humphries, G. and McConnell, H.,** Antigen mobility in membranes and complement-mediated immune attack, *Proc. Nat. Acad. Sci. U.S.A.,* 72, 2483, 1975.
68. **de Gier, J., Mandersloot, J., and van Deenen, L.,** Lipid composition and permeability of liposomes, *Biochim. Biophys. Acta,* 150, 666, 1968.
69. **Kroes, J. and Ostwald, R.,** Erythrocyte membranes. Effect of increased cholesterol content on permeability, *Biochim. Biophys. Acta,* 249, 647, 1971.
70. **Grunze, M. and Deuticke, B.,** Changes of membrane permeability due to extensive cholesterol depletion in mammalian erythrocytes, *Biochim. Biophys. Acta,* 356, 125, 1974.
71. **Norman, A., Demel, R., de Kruyff, B., Geurts van Kessel, W., and van Deenen, L.,** Studies on the biological properties of polyene antibiotics. Comparison of other polyenes with Filipin in their ability to interact specifically with sterol, *Biochim. Biophys. Acta,* 290, 1, 1972.
72. **Aswad, C. and Ostwald, R.,** Spiculated erythrocytes of cholesterol-fed guinea pigs. Changes of morphology, composition and osmotic fragility, *Proc. Soc. Exp. Biol. Med.,* 153, 505, 1976.

73. **Cooper, R., Arner, E., Wiley, J., and Shattil, S.,** Modification of red cell membrane structure by cholesterol-rich dispersions, *J. Clin. Invest.*, 55, 115, 1975.
74. **Forstner, G., Sabesin, S., and Isselbacher, K.,** Rat intestinal microvillus membranes, *Biochem. J.*, 106, 381, 1968.
75. **Coleman, R.,** Membrane bound enzymes and membrane ultrastructure, *Biochim. Biophys. Acta*, 300, 1, 1973.
76. **Grisham, C. and Barnett, R.,** Role of lipid phase transitions in the regulation of the ($Na^+ + K^+$) adenosine triphosphatase, *Biochemistry*, 12, 2635, 1973.
77. **Zeylemaker, W., Jansen, H., Veeger, C., and Slater, E.,** Studies on succinate dehydrogenase. VII. The effect of temperature on succinate oxidation, *Biochim. Biophys. Acta*, 242, 14, 1971.
78. **Bloj, B., Morero, R., Farias, R., and Trucco, R.,** Membrane lipid fatty acids and regulation of membrane bound enzymes, *Biochim. Biophys. Acta*, 311, 67, 1973.
79. **Kimelberg, H. and Papahadjopoulos, D.,** Effects of phospholipid acyl chain fluidity, phase transitions and cholesterol on ($Na^+ + K^+$)-stimulated adenosine-triphosphatase, *J. Biol. Chem.*, 249, 1071, 1974.
80. **Stuart, M. J., Gerrard, J., and White, J.,** Effect of cholesterol on production of thromboxane B_2 by platelets in vitro, *N. Engl. J. Med.*, 302, 6, 1980.
81. **Sandermann, H.,** Regulation of membrane enzymes by lipids, *Biochim. Biophys. Acta*, 515, 209, 1978.
82. **Brulet, P. and McConnell, H.,** Structural and dynamical aspects of membrane immunochemistry using model membranes, *Biochemistry*, 16, 1209, 1977.
83. **Inbar, M. and Shinitzky, M.,** Cholesterol as a bioregulator in the development and inhibition of leukemia, *Proc. Nat. Acad. Sci. U.S.A.*, 71, 4229, 1974.
84. **Borochov, H. and Shinitzky, M.,** Vertical displacement of membrane proteins indicated by changes in microviscosity, *Proc. Nat. Acad. Sci. U.S.A.*, 73, 4526, 1976.
85. **Rivnay, B., Globerson, A., and Shinitzky, M.,** Perturbation of lymphocyte response to concanavalin A by exogenous cholesterol and lecithin, *Eur. J. Immunol.*, 8, 185, 1978.
86. **Kandutsch, A. and Chen, H.,** Consequences of blocked sterol synthesis in cultured cells. DNA synthesis and membrane composition, *J. Biol. Chem.*, 252, 409, 1977.
87. **Chen, H., Heininger, H-J., and Kandutsch, A.,** Alteration of $^{86}Rb^+$ influx and efflux following depletion of membrane sterol in L cells, *J. Biol. Chem.*, 253, 3180, 1978.
88. **Sinha, A., Shattil, S., and Coleman, R.,** Cyclic AMP metabolism in cholesterol-rich platelets, *J. Biol. Chem.*, 252, 3310, 1977.

Chapter 3

CHOLESTEROL TRANSPORT

Suk Yon Oh

TABLE OF CONTENTS

I. INTRODUCTION

Epidemiological and clinical studies of past decades have shown a correlation between high concentrations of blood cholesterol and an increased risk of having premature cardiovascular disease, which may occur as a result of the formation of atherosclerotic lesions in the arteries. Since the pioneering work of Gofman and his colleagues in the early 1950s, the study of plasma lipoproteins, particularly apolipoproteins in recent years, has significantly broadened our understanding of cholesterol metabolism and cholesterol transport.

Virtually all plasma cholesterol (95%), the second largest serum lipid fraction after phospholipids, is loosely bound to lipoprotein which has evolved to facilitate lipid transport in extracellular fluid. Since it was identified as a constituent of animal food products in 1912, it has become well known that cholesterol is essential to vital cellular functions. In contrast, any excessive amount of the water insoluble sterol can cause adverse effects such as development of atherosclerosis and other blood vessel diseases. Thus, mammalian cells are faced with the dual problem of providing sufficient cholesterol for functions and, at the same time, of preventing excess accumulation of sterol.

A consideration of cholesterol transport among organs should address itself to those features of cholesterol transport known or suspected to be relevant to the clinical manifestation of coronary artery diseases, which are the leading cause of death in this country.

II. LIPOPROTEINS AS TRANSPORT VEHICLES

Lipoproteins are specialized systems which serve to solubilize and transport cholesterol, triglycerides, and phospholipids, otherwise water insoluble substances, through plasma from sites of lipid absorption and synthesis to sites of storage and utilization. Lipoproteins are composed of lipids and proteins, and can be considered as a linear spectrum of discrete and finite particles with a changing pattern of lipid and protein composition.

The physical characteristics of lipoproteins are related to their lipid content and composition. The flotation properties of lipoproteins are a direct function of the relative ratio of lipid to protein. Plasma lipoproteins have been conventionally classified into four major families according to their size and density.[1,2] Using centrifugal force to float them on each density, these are chycomicrons, very low density lipoproteins (VLDL), low density lipoproteins (LDL), and high density lipoproteins (HDL). Lipoproteins are constructed with the proteins and phospholipids as charged polar molecules on the surface and the nonpolar molecules, such as triglycerides and cholesteryl esters inside of the molecules. Accordingly, these lipidprotein complexes have remarkable hydrophilic properties in spite of a lipid content that may be as high as 99% by weight.

Lipoproteins are also classified as nonmigrating (chylomicron), beta (LDL), prebeta (VLDL), and alpha lipoprotein (HDL) by electrophoretic mobility of lipoproteins along with alpha and beta globulins on serum protein electrophoresis.[3] Ultracentrifugation (S_f) and electrophoresis are the two major techniques employed to characterize and measure lipoproteins because of their nondestructive nature. These two systems of nomenclature, therefore, can usually be considered essentially exchangeable. Chylomicron and VLDL are primarily glyceride carriers while LDL and HDL carry most of the blood cholesterol. A detailed discussion of the composition and structure of plasma lipoproteins is beyond the objective and scope of this paper. These have been well described in several recent reviews.[4-6]

Chylomicrons and VLDL have been termed the micellar lipoproteins by Schumaker and Adams[7] in distinction to pseudomolecular lipoproteins found in the LDL and HDL classes. Chylomicrons are formed in the small intestine during active fat absorption and serve to transport dietary triglycerides from the intestine to the plasma and ultimately to sites of utilization in the tissues. These esters represent the bulk of lipid cargo transferred through plasma in the course of a day.

Chylomicrons are the largest and lightest of the lipid transport particles of alimentary origin with physical properties of: hydrated density, 0.95 g/ml; flotation rate (S_f), 400; molecular weight, 10^3 to 10^4 million; diameter, 5000Å; shape, spherical; electrophoretic mobility, nonmigrating. They are composed of, by weight, approximately 80% to 95% triglyceride.[6] Less than 2% of chylomicron composition is due to protein. Apoprotein B and C constitute about 90% of the total protein moiety of chylomicrons. Apo A-I and A-II account for about 12% of the apoprotein content of chylomicrons isolated from human thoracic duct lymph.[8,9] Apo A-I has been identified, however, as a major apoprotein of rat mesenteric lymph chylomicrons[10] and has been reported to comprise 30% of their apoprotein mass.[11] A small amount of the arginine rich peptide (apoprotein E), approximately 4% of the total protein mass, is also found in chylomicrons.[12] After exposure to serum lipoproteins, the content of apo-E and apo-C in rat mesenteric lymph chylomicrons increases, while A-I content decreases.[12]

The VLDL share many structural features with chylomicrons though their metabolic functions differ in fundamentals. Both of them are primarily triglyceride carriers from liver and intestine to internal tissues. It has been shown that, unlike chylomicrons, VLDL are synthesized and secreted by both the liver and the intestinal mucosal cells.[13,14] Intestinal and hepatic VLDL, however, differ at least initially in regard to peptide composition.

The VLDL is separable by ultracentrifugation at $d < 1.006$ g/mℓ and has a flotation rate of S_f 20 to 400. This lipoprotein fraction is composed of about 50 to 60% triglycerides, 18 to 20% phospholipids, 10 to 12% unesterified cholesterol, 4 to 6% esterified cholsterol, and 8 to 12% protein.[15] VLDL is visualized as being spherical particles with variable sizes 300 to 900Å by electronmicroscopy with negative staining technique. Its molecular weight ranges from 5 to 10 million.[2] In contrast to chylomicrons, S_f 20 to 400 lipoproteins appear to transport endogenous glycerides of liver and intestine.[16] The VLDL apoprotein represents a mixture of apo A, apo B, apo C, and apo E, and their relative content are trace amounts, 40%, 40 to 80%, and 13%, respectively.[5]

In human plasma, LDL is the major cholesterol carrying vehicle. About 50% of the LDL mass is cholesterol, predominantly in the esterified form (greater than 70%); protein and phospholipids comprise about 20 to 25% each of the total mass. Triglycerides account for the remaining few percent of the particle mass. The mean diameter by negative staining is 220A (ranging from 170 to 260) with molecular weight of 2.2×10^6.[17] The plasma LDL fraction is conventionally isolated in the preparative ultracentrifuge by flotation between the density 1.006 to 1.063 g/mℓ and has a flotation rate (S_f) of 0 to 20. The major apoprotein present in LDL is apo B along with small quantities of C-apoproteins.[18] The number of apoprotein B subunits in LDL is unknown but estimated to range between 2 and 60.[19,20] The origin of LDL is uncertain, but most or all of plasma LDL may be derived from the catabolism of VLDL.

The composition and metabolism of high density lipoprotein (HDL) have recently become subjects of increasing interest, largely due to the finding that HDL cholesterol is inversely correlated with the incidence of coronary artery disease. Human HDL, isolated by ultracentrifugation in the density range of 1.063 to 1.21 g/mℓ from plasma, is composed of about 50% protein, 25 to 30% phospholipids, 20% cholesterol, and 5% triglyceride.[6,15] The protein moiety of HDL consists of apolipoprotein A-I, A-II, B, C-I, C-II, C-III, D, E, and F.[5,21] Among them, apo A-I and apo A-II comprise about 90% of HDL protein with an apo A-I/apo A-II weight ratio of ca. 3:1. HDL are conventionally divided into the two major subclasses: HDL_2 (d,1.062 to 1.125 g/mℓ) and HDL_3 (d,1.25 to 1.21 g/mℓ).[22] HDL_2 is composed of ca. 55% lipid and 45% protein, while 55% of HDL_3 mass is due to protein.[15,23] HDL_2 has a mean molecular weight of 360,000 and atom and particle diameter of 100 to 150Å. The mean molecular weight of HDL_3 is 175,000 and the particle diameter ranges from 65 to 95Å.[21] Anderson et al.[24] have separated two discernible migrating HDL subfractions into HDL_{2a} and HDL_{2b} (molar ratio, 2:1) by analytical ultracentrifugation, preceded by a preparative ultracentrifugal separation of HDL_2. Their data for the levels of HDL_{2a} and HDL_{2b} in relation to those of total HDL or HDL_3 indicated that HDL_3 may be a precursor of HDL_{2a} and HDL_{2b} upon loading with phospholipids and cholesterol. Several other isolation procedures such as electrophoresis-heparin affinity chromatography column, heparin-Mn^{++} precipitation, zonal rotar, and agarose column chromatography have been developed for isolation of lipoprotein families from HDL. Regardless of the manner of isolation, however, HDL do not consist of a single macromolecular complex but represent a mixture of several discrete lipoprotein families. Alaupovic, et al.[25] found the very high density lipoprotein (VHDL) at a density greater than that of HDL_3 but less than that of the infranatant fraction (1.21 < d < 1.25 g/mℓ). The infranatant fraction of ultracentrifugation (d > 1.21 g/mℓ) contains 9 to 12% of plasma apo A-I[26] and a significant amount of apo A-I was reported in the d > 1.21 g/mℓ ultracentrifugal residue.[27] It is generally known that the shear-dependent denaturation during ultracentrifugal procedures alters the characteristics of particles and results in apoprotein diffusibility (particularly apo Cs and E) and heterogeneity of HDL subclasses.

Another HDL subclass is LP(a) lipoprotein (sinking pre-B lipoprotein), found in varying amounts in human plasma in the density range 1.055 to 1.085 g/mℓ.[28] This lipoprotein is composed of ca. 27% protein, 65% lipid, and 8% carbohydrate. Its major apoproteins are apo-B (about 65%) and possibly albumin.[29] The major lipids are cholesterol (mainly esterified) and phospholipids. The routes of synthesis and catabolism of the LP(a) lipoprotein are not yet known, nor is its physiological significance.

The metabolic functions of HDL are unknown, but available information suggests the HDL may play roles in triglyceride clearance[28] and in cholesterol esterification in plasma as the natural substrate for lecithin-cholesterol acyltransferase (LCAT).[29] In connection with the former function, it serves as the activator protein for lipoprotein lipase[30] and for the latter role, apo A-I and C-I function as cofactors for LCAT activity. Recent evidence indicates that HDL plays a role in removal of cholesterol from peripheral tissues as a reverse transport vehicle. This HDL function will be discussed in detail in a later section.

III. CHOLESTEROL ABSORPTION FROM INTESTINE

The lymphatic transport of cholesterol is of great quantitative importance in the overall metabolism of cholesterol. The potential importance of the intestine in cholesterol transport lies in the fact that it is the sole extrahepatic site of plasma lipoprotein synthesis, and it is the initial portal entry for the absorbed cholesterol along with other wide varieties of compounds. It is now well established that exogenous cholesterol is absorbed almost exclusively by way of the intestinal lymph as chylomicrons.[31]

The absorption of cholesterol is one of two sources for new sterol in animals and man along with cholesterol synthesis. Cholesterol within the intestinal lumen consists of a mixture of exogenous (dietary) and endogenous origin of both free and esterified forms. The endogenous cholesterol is chiefly derived from biliary sterols and sterols from other intestinal secretion and from desquamation of intestinal mucosal cells.[32]

The first step of the cholesterol absorption process is hydrolysis of dietary cholesteryl esters to free cholesterol by pancreatic cholesteryl ester hydrolase.[33] In the subsequent steps, the intraluminal free cholesterol in the presence of sufficient concentrations of bile acids and other amphipathic substances such as monoglycerides and free fatty acids is solubilized in mixed micelles and absorbed by the intestinal mucosal epithelial cells across the cell membrane of the brush border by passive diffusion. The absorbed free cholesterol mixes with an intracellular pool of unesterified cholesterol from, in part, *de novo* synthesis. A major portion of this pool is next esterified with long chain fatty acids by cholesterol esterase in the absorptive cell. The cholesteryl esters are then incorporated into chylomicron particles along with triglycerides, phospholipids, free cholesterol, and specific apoproteins. The lipoprotein particles are initially assembled within the apical smooth endoplasmic reticulum,[34] and subsequently accumulate in the Golgi apparatus to be discharged into the lateral intracellular spaces.

Cage and Fish[35] designated the lipoproteins produced by the intestine after a fatty meal as "chylomicrons." It has been assumed that the nonpolar lipids (triglyceride and cholesteryl ester) are carried within the hydrophobic core of the particles while the polar components, protein, phospholipid, and free cholesterol which are capable of stable interaction with water are exterior to such a hydrophobic interior,[36] which is analogous to a micellar structure.

The precise mechanism for the assembly and secretion of chylomicrons remains unknown, but data obtained from human abetalipoproteinemia subects and animal experiments with protein synthesis inhibitors have inferred an obligatory role for the apoprotein in this process.[37] The hereditary defect in B-apoprotein biosynthesis (abetaliproteinemia) results in a marked impairment of chylomicron secretion and an accumulation of triglyceride within the mucosal epithelial cells. Windmueller et al.[38] and Havel et al.[39] showed that impaired chylomicron secretion accompanied by intracellular triglyceride accumulation has been produced experimentally in rats treated with protein synthesis inhibitors. These data indicate that the rate limiting step for cholesterol absorption across the mucosal cell membrane into the lymph is the availability of specific apoproteins within the rough endoplasmic reticulum where the chylomicron particles are assembled. The recent studies of Glickman et al.[40] and Imaizumi et al.[12] unequivocally showed that inhibition of protein synthesis not only impaired fat absorption but, in addition, led to impaired formation of chylomicrons. Thus, proteins play a crucial role in the lipoprotein transport of lipids absorbed from the intestine.

At present, there are three general means for the assessment of cholesterol absorption: the isotopic balance technique,[41] the chemical balance method,[42] and a combination of the two methods.[43] All these three methods, however, are limited to give net absorption. Recently, Zilversmit[44] introduced the dual isotope tracer method to measure cholesterol absorption. There is, at this time, no means for assessing the magnitude of enterohepatic and enterolymphatic circulation of cholesterol. (See Chapter 5 for further discussion of this problem.) In abetaliproteinemia, the patients are unable to form chylomicrons after a fatty meal; accordingly, triglyceride accumulates in the intestinal absorptive cells and fat malabsorption results. Despite these disabilitics, they suffer only mild fat malabsorption[37] implying the existence of an alternate pathway, i.e., direct entry into the portal vein. Such a pathway has been known to occur to a limited extent in normal animals and in conditions in which intestinal protein synthesis and chylomicron formation is inhibited.[45]

IV. LIPOPROTEIN METABOLISM

A. Chylomicrons

All chylomicrons and some VLDL, bound in plasma, are synthesized within the endoplasmic reticulum of the intestinal mucosal cells. Chylomicrons, after eventually entering the circulation via the lymphatics, are recognized and metabolized by clearing factor, a heparin-activated lipoprotein lipase (triacylglycerol acylhydrolase), situated on the capillary endothelium of extrahepatic tissues.[46] The triglycerides in association with the chylomicrons cause the plasma of many animal species to become markedly turbid. When heparin is administered into such blood the turbidity of the plasma prepared from the post heparin blood is completely cleared.[47] This clearing reaction is due to the hydrolysis of triglyceride of the chylomicrons by a lipase which is released into the blood following the heparin injection. This lipase has been named clearing factor or lipoprotein lipase (LPL).[48] The degradation of chylomicrons yields free fatty acids and glycerides producing remnant particles which are smaller than the nascent chylomicrons and have an altered lipid composition.[49] The free fatty acids released by the action of the lipoprotein lipase combine with plasma albumin and the plasma becomes clear due to the solubility of the free fatty acid-albumin complex.[50] The lipoprotein lipase is believed to be present at the surface of the capillary endothelial cells. LPL is known as the control enzyme for the hydrolysis of triglycerides and cellular uptake as free fatty acids and 2-monoglyceride fatty acids during the absorption of a fatty meal. The rate of uptake of fatty acids liberated by LPL is very rapid in adipose and muscle tissue. In rat, more than 80% of the labeled triglyceride fatty acids are recovered in adipose and muscle, and only 20% in other tissues, principally the liver, within a few minutes.

At least two different lipases are found in post heparin plasma from different tissue origin: one is of adipose tissue origin whereas the other originates in the liver.[51] In type I hyperlipoproteinemia, a complete absence of extrahepatic triglyceride lipase is characteristic and the activity of the liver enzyme seems to be present at "normal" levels.[52] It has also been shown that the two enzymes have different functional roles during the process of intravascular triglyceride hydrolysis in that the liver enzyme has only limited capacity for hydrolyzing significant amounts of triglyceride from intact glyceride-laden lipoprotein.[53,54] There are post heparin lipoprotein lipases which exhibit distinct activities toward diglycerides and monoglycerides.[55-57]

There is evidence that endogenous heparin, or a closely related substance, forms an integral part of the enzyme as it exists in the tissues[53] and that functionally it may be concerned both in the combination of the enzyme with its substrate and in preventing its inactivation. Endogenous heparin may also be responsible for binding the clearing factor lipase at the capillary wall. For the normal activity of triglyceride hydrolysis by lipoprotein lipases, a specific protein cofactor is necessary. Apo C-II is the cofactor protein for full enzyme activity. Apo C-I has also been reported to activate a specific lipoprotein lipase[30] while apo C-III may inhibit the enzyme activity.[58]

Felts and Mayes[59] have shown that remnant particles of chylomicrons produced by lipoprotein lipase action contain firmly bound LPL, and that neither chylomicrons nor VLDL without binding to LPL are recognized by liver as a substrate suggesting that the LPL attached to the remnants is the signal that allows the liver to recognize the remnants. The cholesteryl esters in chylomicron remnants are taken up predominantly by the liver[60] after which they are slowly hydrolyzed to free cholesterol and free fatty acids. There is a delay of several hours as the liver rearranges hepatic cholesterol of two origins, dietary and endogenous, with the sterols of blood and other tissue.[61] The rate of the reassembling process for VLDL or LDL may depend on the availability of various components of the particles, notably the apoproteins. The 1980 model of apo B metabolism indeed revealed a delay of apo B biosynthesis in liver or gut cell[62] for the secretion of apo B into plasma may require coupling of the apoprotein with availability of triglyceride in the golgi apparatus of the hepatocyte or gut cells.

B. Very Low Density Lipoproteins

The functional difference between the two triglyceride carriers would be that the chylomicrons are associated with the transport of dietary fat absorbed through the intestinal mucosal cells while the intestinal VLDL carry endogenous lipids similar to the liver VLDL.

VLDL is the primary lipoprotein class, synthesized and secreted by the intestine and liver as the precurser of plasma VLDL. Nascent VLDL lacks C apoproteins,[63] and picks them up in plasma while undergoing stepwise delipidation mediated by lipoprotein lipase. There is, however, difference between intestinal lymph and hepatic VLDL, at least initially, in regard to peptide composition. Intestinal VLDL, although they migrate electrophoretically to the pre-B region, nevertheless are slower than plasma VLDL. If lymph VLDL first are mixed with VLDL-free serum and then are immediately subject to electrophoresis, their mobility is identical to that of plasma VLDL, implying that their surface charge has increased, presumably as a result of the adsorption of additional peptides.[64] Experiments with isolated perfused rat liver and intestine have shown that very little, if any, apo C is secreted with newly synthesized VLDL and HDL by the perfused intestine while both VLDL and HDL isolated from liver perfusate definitely contain apo C. Therefore, once entered into plasma, the intestinal lymph VLDL are apparently metabolized by the same mechanisms as are hepatic VLDL. It is not clear whether the newly synthesized apo C secreted from the liver first enters VLDL or HDL. Hamilton[14] has presented evidence to support HDL as the major first entry site for apo C. The presence of apo C in the plasma of patients with either abetalipoproteinemia of familial HDL deficiency (Tangier disease)[65,66] suggest that apo C metabolism is independent of that of apo B and apo A.

Experimental evidences have shown that significant quantities of plasma VLDL are of intestinal origin. A metabolic turnover study showed 20 to 40% of the total plasma VLDL is attributable to the intestine.[64] The intestinal synthesis of VLDL is known to be varied depending on the type of diet. High carbohydrate diet[67] or ethanol administration[68] increase the triglyceride synthesis in intestinal mucosal cells resulting in high endogenous VLDL production. Fatty acid composition of diet may be an important determinant of the physical properties of the triglyceride-rich lipoproteins secreted by both the intestine and the liver. With unsaturated fat lymph lipoprotein particles are of a size and density range typical for chylomicrons (800A, S_f 400), whereas with saturated fat they resemble typical VLDL.[69]

There is a precursor-product relationship between VLDL-B and LDL-B, and during lipolysis, apo Cs and apo E are removed and shuttled to HDL mainly, but also to LDL and 1.21 bottom.

C. Low Density Lipoproteins

Following enzymatic hydrolysis of VLDL triglycerides in vitro, a net production of LDL particles was reported.[70] Consistent with such a finding is the observation that heparin injection in vivo leads to a decreased concentration of plasma VLDL and a concomitant increase of plasma LDL,[71] and that in Type 1 hyperlipoproteinemia there is a low concentration of LDL.[72]

Several metabolic studies utilizing apoprotein labeling techniques have also shown that VLDL is at least partially metabolized to LDL.[73-77] Studies with iodinated VLDL and iodinated apo B in VLDL[73] revealed that VLDL is initially catabolized to the intermediate density lipoproteins (IDL, S_f 20 to 60) and later to LDL. In the kinetic studies of apoproteins B and C in normal and hyperlipoproteinemic subjects, Berman et al.[78] demonstrated that the VLDL particles undergo a series of density increments during a number of delipidation steps (triglyceride hydrolysis), during which apo B stays with the particle until the density reaches an intermediate density lipoprotein (IDL) range. In their normal human subjects, all IDL apo B eventually became LDL. The apo C was lost during the VLDL delipidation and apo C lost by VLDL and IDL was recycled to HDL, and most of it was then picked up by newly synthesized VLDL.

The liver has been believed to be the major site for cholesterol breakdown and the assumption that the liver would be the major site of LDL removal from the plasma was supported by a conclusion drawn from studies in rats.[79] Hays et al.,[80] following the fate of ^{125}I-LDL, have also reported that in the rat the liver is a major site of LDL catabolism. Sniderman et al.,[81] however, demonstrated that the extrahepatic tissues are the chief sites for LDL catabolism. They compared the disappearance of ^{125}I-labeled LDL from plasma in intact and in hepatectomized swine and found that the rate of irreversible removal of LDL from plasma was increased rather than decreased by hepatectomy, indicating that the liver is not the major site for LDL removal.

During the last five years, Drs. Brown and Goldstein[82] at the University of Texas elegantly elucidated the receptor mediated control of LDL catabolism in cultured human fibroblasts. The pathway by which LDL is metabolized in cultured human fibroblasts is as follows: The initial event involves the binding of LDL to receptors with high and specific binding affinity. The LDL receptors bind only those human plasma lipoproteins that contain apoprotein B, that is mainly LDL. In order for LDL to be catabolized, the LDL that is bound to the receptor enters the cell in a process that resembles absorptive endocytosis. The internalized LDL is assimilated into endocytotic vesicles (endosomes) that fuse with lysosomes in which LDL apoprotein is rapidly hydrolyzed to free amino acids then released into the culture medium. Lysosomal acid lipase hydrolyzes cholesteryl esters of LDL and the resultant free cholesterol is chiefly transferred to the cellular membranes. The accumulation of free cholesterol within the cell suppresses 3-hydroxy-3-methylglutaryl/coenzyme A reductase (HMG CoA reductase), causing a reduction of cholesterol synthesis and simultaneously activates an acyl-CoAolesteryl acyltransferase (ACAT), facilitating its own reesterification. The endogenously reesterified cholesterol is preferentially esterified with oleic and palmitoleic acids, in contrast to the plasma cholesteryl esters which are esterified with polyunsaturated fatty acids by lecithin-cholesterol acyl transferase (LCAT).

The overall process of the LDL receptor-mediated interaction of LDL with cells is to transfer free and esterified cholesterol from plasma LDL to the peripheral cells. Goldstein and Brown also demonstrated the presence of feedback regulation of the LDL receptor in the cell to regulate the activity of the LDL receptor. The mutant cells of the homozygous familial hypercholesterolemia patient lacks the LDL receptor, therefore fails to bind and internalize LDL. Consequently, there would never be an appreciable amount of exogenous cholesterol from LDL within the cell, with the result that the unsuppressed HMG CoA reductase keeps synthesizing cholesterol to the extent that cholesterol accumulates to the level of hypercholesterolemia. From these observations, it is apparent that receptor-mediated LDL catabolism in cultured cells explains the in vivo observations of Steinberg and coworkers[81] who reported that nonhepatic tissues are the major sites for LDL degradation.

D. High Density Lipoproteins

Synthesis and secretion of HDL is thought to occur in both liver and intestine.[83] This opinion is derived from work showing that the major HDL apoprotein is present in the cell[83] and accumulates in perfusates of these organs.[84] Hamilton et al.[85] used the perfused rat liver to study hepatic synthesis of HDL in the presence of an inhibitor of LCAT enzyme, which is responsible for cholesterol esterification in the plasma, and found that nascent HDL secreted from the perfused rat liver resembled the discoidal HDL that occurs in plasma of patients with genetically determined LCAT deficiency.[86] These disk shaped particles are characterized by a high concentration of arginine-rich peptides and a low concentration of esterified cholesterol like the nascent form of plasma HDL.

Intestinal and liver perfusion studies in the rat indicate that both these organs can synthesize apo A-I, but the liver appears to be the major source of the C-apoproteins and apo E.[87,88] Both apo A-I and apo A-II have been localized in human jejunal epithelial cells by immunochemical techniques.[89,90] Compositional study of mesenteric lymph chylomicrons in the rat showed that the proteins of chylomicrons from intestine resemble those of serum HDL, and are substantially different from those of VLDL of blood serum.[91] Protein composition analysis of mesenteric lymph chylomicrons of rat revealed that in addition to the B-apoprotein and the C-apoproteins, apoprotein A-I and apo E accounted for 31% and 4% of the total mass, respectively. Within plasma, chylomicrons acquire more C-apoproteins from HDL.[92]

The relative contribution of the intestine and the liver to apo A-I, and apo A-II synthesis remain to be established, as do the forms in which lipoproteins containing these apoproteins enter the plasma.[93] Some HDL particles appear to be formed from some of the components of the VLDL and chylomicrons within the circulation.[94,95]

The precise functions of HDL are unknown, but available evidence suggests that HDL plays a role in triglyceride hydrolysis by serving as a reservoir for apoprotein C-II, the cofactor for LPL and may be involved in removal of cholesterol from tissues. HDL is customarily divided into two density classes: HDL_2 (d = 1.063 − 1.125 g/mℓ) and HDL_3 (d = 1.125 − 1.21 g/mℓ). It has been shown that fluctuations in HDL concentrations in serum are mainly due to variations in HDL_2 levels.[96] Anderson et al.[24] reported several interesting findings: an inverse correlation between VLDL and HDL_2, and between LDL and HDL_3, with no correlation between the concentrations of total HDL and HDL_3. They also found that at high concentrations of HDL, there were close amounts of HDL_3, HDL_{2a}, and HDL_{2b} but at lower concentration of total HDL, very small amounts of HDL_{2a}, and HDL_{2b} were detected, which indicates that HDL_3 may be the precursor of HDL_{2a} and HDL_{2b} upon loading with phospholipids and cholesterol.

Mahley and coworkers[97] at NIH have isolated HDL_1 with distinctive biochemical and immunological characteristics from the d = 1.063-1.125 g/mℓ fraction by Geon-Pevikon block electrophoresis. Furthermore, they could separate three additional HDL fractions from HDL_1 (d = 1.063-1.125 g/mℓ) isolated in Geon-Pevikon block electrophoresis by the heparin-sepharose affinity column coupled with $MnCl_2$. By the combination of electrophoresis and heparin affinity chromatography HDL particles containing and lacking apoprotein E were differentiated.

It is apparent that there is heterogeneity in the content of the components in various HDL subclasses with possible distinctive roles. However, it must be accepted that some heterogeneity in HDL has been due to preparative techniques. Any method involving dilution changes the diffusible volume and will result in altered equilibrium and a change in apoprotein composition. Future research in HDL undoubtedly will be directed toward an elucidation of the composition and metabolism of the different HDL subclasses.

The metabolic function of HDL is not clearly understood but recent studies suggest they play a role in cholesterol removal from peripheral tissues to liver. HDL, as physiological substrate and cofactor for lecithin-cholesterol acyltransferase (LCAT), may play a controlling role in cholesterol transport and metabolism.[74] Apo A-I is the activating factor for lecithin-cholesterol acyltransferase which is responsible for cholesterol esterification in plasma.[29] So may apo A-III and C-I play a role in LCAT activation[98] while apo A-II has been shown to inhibit LCAT activity.[99] However, it is unknown what controls the reactivity of substrates for LCAT and what makes them be dormant. Apo HDL_2 was reported to be a less effective activator than apo HDL_3[77] but others[15] reported that apo HDL, apo HDL_2 and apo HDL_3, at low concentrations, were equally effective as activators and equally potent inhibitors at high levels. The difference of arginine rich peptide (ARP) content in HDL_2 and HDL_3 may be related to possible differences among HDL subfractions. This subject remains to be clarified.

The C apoproteins have a significant physiological function in fat transport. Apo C-II together with phospholipid acts as a cofactor for lipoprotein lipase[30] and apo C-III has been reported to inhibit lipoprotein lipase.[100] In contrast to apo A-I, apo A-II is known to be tightly bound to HDL lipids and plays a structural role in the HDL particles.[101] A kinetic study of ^{125}I-HDL in normal human subjects[28] showed that apo A-I and apo A-II are metabolized similarly.

After injection of human ^{125}I-HDL into rats, Eisenberg et al.[102] observed a striking difference in the half-life of apo A-I and apo A-II and also found that apo A-I and A-II are catabolized independetly. Shepherd et al.[103] conducted a kinetic study of apo A-I and A-II in human plasma and found that the catabolic rate of exogenously labeled A-I was concomitantly faster than that of endogenous A-I. Conversely. endogenously and exogenously labeled A-II were catabolized at identical rates, suggesting there is a subpopulation of apo A-I in the lipoprotein particle. The A-I/A-II ratio was significantly related to HDL cholesterol.[104] In Tangier disease, the ratio of apo A-I to apo A-II in HDL particles is 1:3[105] which is exactly opposite to the normal ratio. Thus, it appears that interaction of apo A-I and A-II may be of special importance in the HDL molecule.

V. CHOLESTEROL CONCENTRATIONS IN TISSUES

It has been shown that the bulk of plasma cholesterol is delivered to the extrahepatic tissues by LDL mediated by LDL receptors.[82] Thus far, the LDL receptor has been identified functionally in several cell types examined in culture, including human aortic smooth muscle cells,[106] cultured human lymphocytes,[107] HeLa cells,[82] mouse L-cells,[82] endothelial cells,[108] adipocytes,[109] as well as human fibroblasts.[82] That this receptor functions in vivo as it does in cultured cells has been suggested by other workers.[81,110]

Free cholesterol concentrations in different tissues range from 0.9 mg/g of skeletal muscle to 3.9 mg/g of adrenal gland of wet human tissue.[111] The free cholesterol of organ tissues ranges between 7.1 and 17.8% except for adrenal cholesterol in which the ester form is approximately 83% of the total.[112] About 70% of serum cholesterol is normally esterified.[113]

Studies on the compartmentation of lipid adipose cells by Farkas et al.[114] showed that fat tissue is a major cholesterol storage organ. Adipose tissue was shown to contain 0.6-1.6 mg of cholesterol per gram wet weight. When expressed per unit of protein or organ mass, fat tissue contains a higher concentration of cholesterol than muscle, liver, kidney, or membrane. This means that adipose tissue contained at least one half the amount of cholesterol found in muscle. Furthermore, with growth, the cholesterol concentration in fat tissue per milligram of protein increased selectively compared with liver, kidney, and muscle which remained relatively constant.

Hirsch and Han[115] observed that growth of adipose tissue in rat after birth till age 15 weeks occurs by hyperplasia of fat cells and thereafter primarily by an increase in cell size. It appears that compartmentation of cholesterol at the subcellular level is affected by age. In cells of 150 g rats, one half the cholesterol was associated with the storage droplet and the remainder was structural, in contrast to fat cells from mature rats where 87% of cell cholesterol was in the storage pool.

VI. REVERSE CHOLESTEROL TRANSPORT

A seeming paradox in cholesterol metabolism is that LDL, which carries the bulk of serum cholesterol, is taken up and degraded primarily by peripheral tissues,[81] and that most of the cholesterol can only be broken down and/or excreted to any significant extent via the liver. To explain this paradox, reverse cholesterol transport is rationalized. Cholesterol must necessarily be transported from peripheral sites back to the liver for its eventual degradation and excretion, thus balancing the body's cholesterol content.

Certain lipoproteins may play an important role in cholesterol transport from peripheral tissues to the liver. A hypothesis initially postulated by John Glomset[116] is that HDL is involved in cholesterol transport from the peripheral tissues to the liver, and this is supported by observations in patients with familial HDL deficiency (Tangier disease) who accumulate cholesteryl ester in reticuloendothelial cells throughout the body.[117] More recently, Miller and Miller[118] have proposed that the transport of cholesterol from peripheral tissues to the liver, for subsequent catabolism and excretion, may be a function of plasma HDL.

The demonstration that HDL cholesterol concentration is negatively correlated with the mass of both the rapidly and slowly exchanging pools of body cholesterol supports in vitro evidence for a role of HDL in tissue cholesterol removal.[119] According to Olga and Yechezkiel Stein[120] of Hebrew University-Hadassah Medical School in Jerusalem, HDL can remove cholesterol from a variety of cell types, in vitro. When isotopically labeled cholesterol was incorporated into the adipose tissue of subjects who then lost weight by a low calorie diet, all the labeled cholesterol was recovered in the HDL fraction.[121] It also appears that HDL may block cellular deposition of LDL cholesterol into cells due to competitive binding on the LDL receptors on the cell surface, a necessary first step for accumulation of LDL cholesterol.[122]

The cholesterol efflux out of cells may be accomplished by nascent HDL which is newly synthesized, cholesterol-poor HDL. It has been shown that the discoidal HDL picks up cholesterol from the cell membranes in circulation, during which process the HDL becomes spherical with structural rearrangement by cholesterol esterification by LCAT enzyme.[86]

It has been suggested that newly synthesized cholesterol is a preferred precursor for hepatic bile acid synthesis.[123] This conclusion was drawn based on the observations that the specific radioactivity of 7-hydroxycholesterol was higher than that of cholesterol after incubation of labeled mevalonate with the 10,000xg supernatant fluid of rat liver homogenate.[124] Swartz et al.[125,126] have shown that there are definitive hepatic cholesterol precursor sites associated with the synthesis of bile acids and the secretion of biliary cholesterol. They reported that these sites derive a substantial proportion (70%) of their cholesterol from the plasma in which 60% of this cholesterol is unesterified and 10% is esterified after hydrolysis by the liver cholesteryl ester hydrolase. In studies with a patient with a bile fistula, the authors observed that the free labeled cholesterol from high density lipoproteins was more rapidly incorporated into biliary cholesterol than the free cholesterol from low density lipoproteins. These findings indicate that the liver in man selectively utilizes and secretes the free cholesterol from the high density lipoprotein, supporting the current concept that HDL plays the postulated role as the reverse cholesterol transport vehicle from the peripheral tissues to the liver.

Until recently, cardiologists thought that atherosclerosis was a one-way process, and that once fatty deposits formed in arteries, they could never be cleared away by anything but surgery. Some new studies, however, have found evidence that a combination of diet, exercise, and cholesterol-lowering drugs can reverse atherosclerosis.[127] As to the nature of the reverse cholesterol transport vehicle, evidence indicates that HDL does function to remove cholesterol from peripheral tissues to the liver.[119-123] However, no direct evidence has been obtained in vivo to support the postulated role of HDL as a carrier of cholesterol from the tissues to the liver in man. Bondjers and Bjorkerud[128] have provided experimental evidence in vitro that HDL is indeed capable of promoting efflux of cholesterol out of atherosclerotic arterial tissue.

There is some conflicting information against HDL as the reverse cholesterol transport vehicle. It has been shown that cholesteryl esters of HDL formed by LCAT were transferred to VLDL which eventually ended up to LDL.[129] If this recycling were true, HDL would increase the risk of heart disease instead of having a protective effect. Therefore, the question to be answered is whether elevated HDL cholesterol levels directly prevent cholesterol buildup in arteries as postulated. At this time, reverse cholesterol transport is still a hypothesis. Substantial effort should be devoted to understand the molecular mechanisms of cholesterol egress so that a measure to activate the system can be found.

VII. CHOLESTEROL ESTERIFICATION AND HYDROLYSIS

The accumulation of cholesteryl esters in the arterial wall is a consistent feature of atherosclerotic lesions.[130-131] Cholesteryl esters are hydrolyzed by cholesterol esterase, which is present in the aorta of various animals, such as the rabbit,[132] rat, monkey,[133] and man.[134] It has been suggested that deposition of cholesteryl ester might be a consequence of a relative deficiency of acid cholesteryl ester hydrolase in rabbit arterial wall lysosomes.[135] It is not clear, however, how cholesterol esterase controls cholesteryl ester deposition in the arterial wall.

Once esterified cholesterol has been hydrolyzed to free cholesterol, it can be taken up by the postulated reverse cholesterol transport vehicle by mass action[136] at the cell membrane surface or by a yet unknown mechanism. Thus, the efflux of cholesterol out of the arterial wall may depend initially upon the hydrolysis of cholesteryl esters deposited in the tissue.

Cholesterol uptake by cells and subsequent cholesterol metabolism have been described in cultured cells by Goldstein and Brown.[106] Only free cholesterol can exit the cell in culture through the membrane.[137] In erythrocytes, unesterified cholesterol readily exchanges with plasma cholesterol[138,139] and many investigators have attempted to determine what proportion of membrane cholesterol participates in this exchange process.[140,141]

Shinomiya et al.[142] found two cholesterol esterases in subcellular fractions of rat arterial wall: an acid cholesterol esterase, mainly present in the lysosome rich fraction, and a neutral cholesterol esterase with an optimum activity at pH 7.5, mainly present in the microsome. The physical state of the substrate such as the ratio of phospholipids or detergents to cholesteryl ester for cholesterol esterase has been shown to be of critical importance for enzyme activity.[143,144] When phospholipid-cholesterol vesicles were used as substrate, the cholesteryl esterase activity was highest with phosphotidyl-choline, suggesting that the deposition of cholesteryl ester might be partially regulated by the quantity and quality of phospholipids in the arterial wall.[142] In fact, increased phospholipid synthesis in the arterial wall is reported to result in increased cholesteryl ester deposition.[145]

It was reported that pancreatic cholesterol esterase systems require trihydroxy bile salts as cofactors in the synthesis or hydrolysis of cholesteryl oleate, and that this cofactor requirement is not related to the detergent properties of the bile salt.[146,147] The authors also found that cholic acid protects cholesterol esterase against proteolytic inactivation. Based on these findings, they postulated that (1) bile salt complexed to the allosteric enzyme at or near the active site, or (2) produced a configurational change in the protein. They also reported formation of insoluble sterolenzyme complexes using various sources of cholesterol esterase.

Cholesteryl ester hydrolytic activity has been reported in a variety of tissues including liver, intestine, pancreas, adrenal, adipose tissue, brain, aorta, red blood cell membrane, skin, fibroblasts, isolated macrophages, and smooth muscle cells.[142-148]

Many investigators have studied arterial cholesteryl ester hydrolases but some of the reports appear to conflict, especially with regard to bile salt dependence and optimal pH.[144,149-156] The pH optima were in all cases close to either pH 4.5 or pH 6.8.[152] In general, the acid cholesteryl ester hydrolase activity was quite constant from tissue to tissue, while the neutral enzyme activity as well as the optimal pH varied greatly in tissues.[152,153] Recently, Sloan and Fredrickson[154] compared cholesteryl ester hydrolase activity of pH 4.0 in aortas, lymph nodes, liver, and spleen from apparently normal postmortem cases and from cases of cholesteryl ester storage disease. The level of hydrolysis activity was much lower in the diseased samples than in the normal subjects.

An extensive study of the cholesteryl esterase of rat brain has been undertaken by Eto and Suzuki.[155] They observed two cholesteryl ester hydrolases, namely acidic cholesteryl esterase, with optimum pH 4.2 and neutral enzyme at pH 6.6. Riddle et al.[152] confirmed two separate hydrolyzing enzymes of cholesteryl esters in cultured human fibroblasts and monkey arterial smooth muscle cells. Subcellular fractionation of human fibroblasts revealed that activities at pH 4.5 and pH 6.8 were concentrated in different fractions, the acidic lysosomal and the polysomal with the neutral pH, respectively.

Early in this century, the activating effect of bile salts on cholesterol esterase was reported by Mueller[156] and Nedswedski.[157] Since then, the activating and the protective effect of bile salts, particularly taurocholate have been confirmed by many investigators.[146,147,158] Eto and Suzuki[155] reported that sodium-taurocholate stimulated the acidic enzyme two- to fourfold and the neutral enzyme (pH 6.6) up to fifteenfold by 4m*M* bile salt. This observation has been confirmed by numerous investigators.[146,147,159-161] Taurocholate has also been shown to protect the hydrolytic cholesterol esterase from inactivation due to proteolytic degradation.[146,148,161]

An energy-independent cholesteryl ester synthetase with a pH optimum of 5.0 has been found in atherosclerotic rabbit intima,[162] and in peritoneal macrophage with a pH optimum of 6.3.[163] A characteristic feature of cholesteryl ester synthetase is its independence from energy donors, in particular from ATP. There is another enzyme, the acyl CoA: cholesterol o-acyltransferase (ACAT) which is found in mammalian tissues. Further characterization of ACAT is necessary in the light of its significance in cellular cholesterol metabolism. Intracellular synthesis of cholesteryl esters in the aorta has been shown to play a role at least as significant as the plasma contribution of cholesteryl esters to the accumulation of cholesteryl esters.[164] There is no available information regarding cofactor requirement of the enzyme. From the available data, it is not clear whether cholesteryl ester synthetase is the same as the enzyme acyl CoA-cholesterol-acyltransferase.

VIII. SUMMARY

Cholesterol is transported within the body by various lipoprotein fractions through lipid-protein interaction. Plasma lipoproteins not only function to solubilize lipids but also contain within their apoprotein structure the specific information that dictates the body sites to which the sterol is to be delivered, the amount of cholesterol carried in the plasma, and the duration of its transport.

The plasma cholesterol represents about 10% of the total body pool of cholesterol. Turnover studies of plasma cholesterol revealed that the plasma cholesterol is in exchange with other tissue cholesterol compartments with different equilibrium rate. Since the sterol ring structure cannot be broken and is excreted primarily by the liver, plasma cholesterol association with various lipoproteins is vital for the homeostatic regulation of whole body cholesterol which influences critically the site of the cholesterol pool in the plasma as well as in the body. Lower density lipoproteins carry the bulk of cholesterol to peripheral tissues where they are taken up as donors of cellular cholesterol. The tissue cholesterol is brought into plasma and transported back to the liver by yet unknown mechanisms possibly by high density lipoproteins as the reverse cholesterol transport vehicle. Enzymatic activity for cholesteryl ester formation in the plasma and cell, and for hydrolysis of the steryl ester, may be factors in regulation of the homeostasis of body cholesterol.

REFERENCES

1. **Havel, R. J., Eder, H. A., and Bragdon, J. H.,** Distribution and chemical composition of ultracentrifugally separated lipoproteins in human sera. *J. Clin. Invest.,* 34, 1345, 1955.
2. **Lindgren, F. T. and Nichols, A. V.,** in *The Plasma Lipoproteins,* Putnam, F. W., Ed., Academic Press, New York, 1960, 1 Vol. 2.
3. **Kunkel, H. G. and Slater, R. J.,** Lipoprotein patterns of serum obtained by zone electrophoresis, *J. Clin. Invest.,* 31, 677, 1952.
4. **Eisenberg, S. and Levy, R. I.,** Lipoprotein metabolism, in *Advances in Lipid Research,* Vol. 13, Paoletti, R. and Dritchevsky, D., Eds. Academic Press, New York, 1975, 2.
5. **Schaefer, E. J., Eisenberg, S., and Levy, R. I.,** Lipoprotein apoprotein metabolism, *J. Lipid Res.,* 19, 667, 1978.
6. **Levy, R. I., Blum, C. B., and Schaefer, E. J.,** in *Liproprotein Metabolism,* Greten, H., Ed., Springer-Verlag, Berlin, 1976, 56.
7. **Schumaker, V. N. and Adams, G. H.,** Circulating liproproteins, *Ann. Rev. Biochem.,* 38, 113, 1969.
8. **Kostner, G. and Holasek, A.,** Characterization and quantification of the apolipoprotein from human chyle chylomicrons, *Biochemistry,* 11, 1217, 1972.
9. **Schaefer, E. J., Jenkins, L. L., and Brewer, H. B., Jr.,** Human chylomicron apolipoprotein metabolism, *Biochem. Biophys. Res. Commun.,* 80, 405, 1978.
10. **Glickman, R. M. and Green, P. H. R.,** The intestine as a source of apolipoprotein A-1, *Proc. Natl. Acad. Sci. U.S.A.,* 74, 2569, 1977.
11. **Fainaru, M., Havel, R. J., and Felker, T. E.,** Radioimmunoassay of apolipoprotein A-1 of rat serum, *Biochim. Biophys. Acta.,* 446, 56, 1976.
12. **Imaizumi, K., Fainaru, M., and Havel, R. J.,** Transfer of apolipoproteins (A-1 and ARP) between rat mesentric lymph chylomicrons and serum lipoproteins, Circulation 54 (Suppl. 11) Abstr. 1976.
13. **Mahley, R. W., Hamilton, R. L., and Lequire, V. S.,** Characterization of lipoprotein particles isolated from the golgi apparatus of rat liver, *J. Lipid Res.* 10, 443, 1969.
14. **Hamilton, R. L.,** Synthesis and secretion of plasma lipoproteins. Pharmacological control of lipid metabolism, *Advan. Exp. Med. Biol.,* 26, 7, 1972.
15. **Margolis, S.,** in *Structural and Functional Aspects of Lipoproteins in Living Systems,* Tria, E., and Scanu, A. M., Eds., 369, Academic Press, London, 1969.
16. **Cornwell, D. G., Kruger, F. A., Hamwi, G. H., and Brown, J.,** Studies on the characterization of human serum lipoproteins separated by ultracentrifugation in a density gradient, *Am. J. Clin. Nutr.,* 9, 24, 1961.
17. **Forte, T. and Nichols, A. V.,** Application of electron microscopy to the study of plasma lipoprotein structure, in *Advances in Lipid Research,* Vol. 10, Paoletti and D. Kritchevsky, Eds., Academic Press, New York. 1972, 1.
18. **Lee, D. M. and Alaupovic, P.,** Physicochemical properties of low density lipoproteins of normal human plasma, *Biochem. J.,* 137, 155, 1974.
19. **Mateu, L., Tardieu, A., Luzzati, V., Aggerbeck, L., and Scanu, A. M.,** On the structure of human serum low density lipoprotein, *J. Mol. Biol.,* 70, 105, 1972.
20. **Smith, R., Dawson, J. R., and Tanford, C.,** The size and number of polypeptide chains in human serum low density lipoprotein, *J. Biol. Chem.,* 247, 3376, 1972.
21. **Schaefer, E. J., Foster, D. M., Jenkins, L. L., Lindgren, F. T., Berman, M., Levy, R. I., and Brewer, H. B., Jr.,** The composition and metabolism of high density lipoprotein subfractions, *Lipids,* 14, 511, 1979.
22. **DeLalla, O. F. and Gofman, J. W.,** Ultracentrifugal analysis of serum lipoproteins, *Methods Biochem. Anal.,* 1, 459, 1954.
23. **Skipski, V. P., in** *Blood Lipids and Lipoproteins. Quantitation, Composition and Metabolism,* Nelson, G. J., Ed., Wiley-Interscience, New York, 521, 1972.

24. **Anderson, D. W., Nichols, A. V., Forte, T. M., and Lindgren, F. T.,** Particle distribution of human serum high density lipoproteins, *Biochim. Biophys. Acta.,* 493, 55, 1977.
25. **Alaupovic, P., Sanbar, S. S., Furman, R. H., Sullivan, M. L., and Walraven, S. L.,** Studies of the composition and structure of serum lipoproteins. Isolation and characterization of very high density lipoproteins of human serum, *Biochemistry,* 5, 4044, 1966.
26. **Schonfeld, G. and Pfleger, B.,** The structure of human high density lipoprotein and the levels of apoprotein A-1 in plasma as determined by radioimmunoassay, *J. Clin. Invest.,* 54, 236, 1974.
27. **Albers, J. J., Wahl, P. W., Cabana, V. G., Hazzard, W. R., and Hoover, J. J.,** Quantification of apoprotein A-1 of human plasma high density lipoprotein, *Metab.,* 25, 633, 1976.
28. **Blum, C. B., Levy, R. I., Eisenberg, S., Hall, M., III, Goebel, R. H., and Berman, M.,** High density lipoprotein metabolism in man, *J. Clin. Invest.,* 60, 795, 1977.
29. **Fielding, C. J., Shore, V. G., and Fielding, P. E,** A protein cofactor of lecithin:cholesterol acyltransferase, *Biochem. Biophys. Res. Commun.,* 46, 1493, 1972.
30. **LaRosa, J. C., Levy, R. I., Herbert, P. N., Lux, S. E., and Fredrickson, D. S.,** A specific apoprotein activator for lipoprotein lipase, *Biochem. Biophys. Res. Commun.,* 41, 57, 1970.
31. **Gangle, A. and Ockner, R. K.,** Intestinal metabolism of lipids and lipoproteins, *Gastroent.,* 68, 167, 1975.
32. **Dietschy, J. M. and Wilson, J. D.,** Regulation of cholesterol metabolism, *New Engl. J. Med.,* 282, 1179, 1970.
33. **Treadwell, C. R. and Vahouny, G. V.,** Cholesterol absorption, in *Handbook of Physiology: A critical, comprehensive presentation of physiological knowledge and concepts, Section 6,* American Physiological Society, Washington, D.C., 1968, 1407.
34. **Cardell, R. R., Jr., Badenhausen, S., and Porter, K. P.,** Intestinal triglyceride absorption in the rat, An electron microscopical study, *J. Cell Biol.,* 34, 123, 1967.
35. **Cage, S. H. and Fish, P. A.,** Fat digestion, absorption, and assimilation in man and animals as determined by the dark-field microscope, and a fat-soluble dye, *Am. J. Anat.,* 34, 1, 1924.
36. **Salpeter, M. M. and Zilversmit, D. B.,** The surface coat of chylomicrons: electron microscopy, *J. Lipid Res.,* 9, 187, 1968.
37. **Ways, P. O., Parmentier, C. M., and Kayden, H. J.,** Studies on the absorptive defect for triglyceride in abetalipoproteinemia, *J. Clin. Invest.,* 46, 35, 1967.
38. **Windmueller, H. G., Herbert, P., and Levy, R. I.,** Biosynthesis of lymph and plasma lipoprotein apoproteins by isolated perfused rat liver and intestine, *J. Lipid Res.,* 14, 215, 1973.
39. **Havel, R. J., Kane, J. P., and Kashyap, M. L.,** Interchange of apoproteins between chylomicrons and high density lipoproteins during alimentary hyperlipemia in man, *J. Clin. Invest.,* 52, 32, 1973.
40. **Glickman, R. M., Kirsch, K., and Isselbacher, K. J.,** Fat absorption during inhibition of protein synthesis: studies of lymph chylomicrons, *J. Clin. Invest.,* 51, 356, 1972.
41. **Wilson, J. D.,** The quantification of cholesterol excretion and degradation in the isotopic steady state in the rat: the influence of dietary cholesterol, *J. Lipid Res.,* 5, 409, 1964.
42. **Miettinen, T. A., Ahrens, E. H., Jr., and Grundy, S. M.,** Quantitative isolation and gas-liquid chromatographic analysis of total dietary and fecal neutral steroids, *J. Lipid Res.,* 6, 411, 1965.
43. **Grundy, S. M. and Ahrend, E. H., Jr.,** An evaluation of relative merits of two ethods for measuring the balance of sterols in man: isotopic balance versus chromatographic analysis, *J. Clin. Invest.,* 45, 1503, 1966.
44. **Zilversmit, D. B.,** A single blood sample dual isotope method for the measurement of cholesterol absorption in rats, *Proc. Soc. Exp. Biol. Med.,* 140, 862, 1972.
45. **Gotto, A. M., Levy, R. I., and John, K.,** On the protein in abetalipoproteinemia, *N. Engl. J. Med.* 284, 813, 1971.
46. **Fielding, C. J.,** Origin and properties of remnant lipoproteins, in *Disturbances in Lipid and Lipoprotein Metabolism,* Dietchy, J. M., Gotto, A. M., Jr., and Ontko, J. A., Eds., Clinical Physiology Series, American Physiological Society, 1977, 83.
47. **Hahn, P. F.,** Abolishment of alimentary lipemia following injection of heparin, *Science,* 98, 19, 1943.
48. **Korn, E. D.,** Clearing factor, a heparin-activated lipoprotein lipase. I. Isolation and characterization of the enzyme from normal rat heart, *J. Biol. Chem.,* 215, 1, 1955.
49. **Redgrave, T. B.,** Formation of cholesterolester-rich particulate lipid during metabolism of chylomicrons, *J. Clin. Invest.,* 49, 465, 1970.
50. **Spector, A. A.,** Fatty acid binding to plasma albumin, *J. Lipid Res.,* 16, 165, 1975.
51. **LaRosa, J. C., Levy, R. I., Windmueller, H. G., and Fredrickson, D. S.,** Comparison of the triglyceride lipase of liver, adipose tissue, and postheparin plasma, *J. Lipid Res.,* 13, 356, 1972.
52. **Krause, R., Levy, R., Windmueller, H., Miller, L., and Fredrickson, D.,** Selective measurement of lipoprotein lipase and hepatic triglyceride lipase in post heparin plasma, *J. Clin. Invest.,* 51, 52a, (Abstract), 1972.

53. **Krause, R. R., Windmueller, H. G., Levy, R. I., and Fredrickson, D. S.,** Selective measurement of two different triglyceride lipase activities in rat postheparin plasma, *J. Lipid Res.*, 14, 286, 1973.
54. **Felts, J. M. and Berry, M. J.,** T he metabolism of free fatty acids and chylomicron triglyceride fatty acids by isolated rat liver cells, *Biochim. Biophys. Acta,* 231, 1, 1971.
55. **Greten, H., Levy, R. I., and Fredrickson, D. S.,** A further characterization of lipoprotein lipase, *Biochim. Biophys. Acta,* 164, 185, 1968.
56. **Nilsson-Ehle, P. and Belfrage, P.,** A monoglyceride hydrolyzing enzyme in human postheparin plasma, *Biochim. Biophys. Acta.*, 270, 60, 1972.
57. **Robinson, D. S.,** Clearing factor lipase and fat transport, *Adv. Lipid Res.*, 1, 133, 1963.
58. **Brown, W. V. and Baginsky, M. L.,** Inhibition of lipoprotein lipase by an apoprotein of human very low density lipoprotein, *Biochem. Biophys. Res. Commun.*, 46, 375, 1972.
59. **Felts, J. M. and Mayes, P. A.,** Lack of uptake and oxidation of chylomicron triglyceride to carbon dioxide and ketone bodies by the perfused rat liver, *Nature,* 206, 195, 1965.
60. **Goodman, D. S.,** The metabolism of chylomicron cholesteryl ester in the rat, *J. Clin. Invest.*, 41, 1886, 1962.
61. **Borgstrom, B., Lindhe, B. A., and Wlodawer, P.,** Absorption and distribution of cholesterol-4-^{14}C in the rat, *Proc. Soc. Exp. Biol.*, 99, 365, 1958.
62. **Fisher, W. R., Zeck, L. A., Barbalaye, P., Warmke, G., and Berman, M.,** Metabolism of apolipoprotein B in subjects with hypertriglyceridemia and polydispersed LDL, *J. Lipid Res.*, In press (personnal communication).
63. **Mahley, R. W., Bennett, B. I., Morre, D. J., Gray, M. E., Thistelwaite, W., and Lequire, V. S.,** Lipoproteins associated with the golgi apparatus isolated from epithelial cells of rat small intestine, *Lab. Invest.*, 25, 435, 1971.
64. **Ockner, R. K., Hughes, F. B., and Isselbach, K. J.,** Very low density lipoproteins of intestinal lymph, *J. Clin. Invest.*, 48, 2079, 1969.
65. **Assman, G., Herbert, P. N., Fredrickson, D. S., and Forte, T.,** Isolation and characterizations of an abnormal high density lipoprotein in Tangier disease, *J. Clin. Invest.*, 60, 242, 1977.
66. **Gotto, A. M., Jr., Levy, R. I., John, K., and Fredrickson, D. S.,** On the protein defect in abetalipoproteinemia, *N. Engl. J. Med.*, 284, 813, 1971.
67. **DenBesten, L., Reyna, R. H., and Conner, W. E.,** The different effects on the serum lipids and fecal steroids of high carbohydrate diets given orally or intravenously, *J. Clin. Invest.*, 52, 1384, 1973.
68. **Mistilis, S. P. and Ockner, R. K.,** Effects of ethanol on endogenous lipid and lipoprotein metabolism in small intestine, *J. Lab. Clin. Med.*, 80, 34, 1972.
69. **Ockner, R. K., Hughes, F. B., and Isselbach, K. J.,** Very low density lipoproteins in intestinal lymph: role in triglyceride and cholesterol transport during fat absorption, *J. Clin. Invest.*, 48, 2367, 1969.
70. **Adams, G. H. and Schumaker, V. N.,** Rapid molecular weight estimates of low density lipoproteins, *Anal. Biochem.*, 29, 117, 1969.
71. **Nichols, A. V., Strisower, E. H., Lindgren, F. T., Adamson, G. L., and Coggiola, E. L.,** Analysis of change in ultracentrifugal lipoprotein profiles following heparin and ethyl-p-chlorophenoxyisobutyrate administration, *Clin. Chim. Acta.*, 20, 277, 1968.
72. **Fredrickson, D. S., Levy, R. I., and Lees, R. S.,** Fat transport in lipoproteins — an integrated approach to mechanisms and disorders, *N. Engl. J. Med.*, 276, 34, 1967.
73. **Bilheimer, D. W., Eisenberg, S., and Levy, R. I.,** The metabolism of very low density lipoproteins. I. Preliminary in vitro and in vivo observations, *Biochim. Biophys. Acta,* 260, 212, 1972.
74. **Reardon, M. F., Fidge, N. H., and Nestle, P. J.,** Catabolism of very low density lipoprotein B apoprotein in man, *J. Clin. Invest.*, 61, 850, 1978.
75. **Eisenberg, S., Bilhemier, D. W., Lindgren, F. T., and Levy, R. I.,** On the metabolis conversion of human plasma very low density lipoproteins, *Biochim. Biophys. Acta,* 326, 361, 1973.
76. **Schonfeld, C., Lees, R. S., George, P. K., and Pfleger, B.,** Assay of total plasma apoliproprotein B concentration in human subjects, *J. Clin. Invest.*, 53, 1458, 1974.
77. **Sigurdsson, G., Nicholl, A., and Lewis, B.,** Conversion of very low density lipoprotein to low density lipoprotein: a metabolic study of apolipoprotein B kinetics in human subjects, *J. Clin. Invest.*, 56, 1481, 1975.
78. **Berman, M., Hall, M., III, Levy, R. I., Eisenberg, S., Bilhemier, D. W., Phair, R. D., and Goebel, R. H.,** Metabolism of apo B and apo C lipoproteins in man: kinetic studies in normal and hyperlipoproteinemic subjects, *J. Lipid Res.*, 19, 38, 1978.
79. **Hotta, S. and Chaikoff, I. L.,** The role of the liver in the turnover of plasma cholesterol, *Arch. Biochem. Biophys.*, 56, 28, 1955.
80. **Hays, R. V., Pottenger, L. A., Reingold, A. L., Getz, G. S., and Wissler, R. W.,** Degradation of I^{125}-labeled serum low density lipoprotein in normal and estrogen treated male rats, *Biochem. Biophys. Res. Commun.*, 44, 1471, 1971.
81. **Sniderman, A. D., Carew, T. E., Chandler, J. G., and Steinberg, D.,** Paradoxical increase in rate of catabolism of low density lipoproteins after hepatectomy, *Science,* 183, 526, 1974.

82. **Brown, M. S., and Goldstein, J. L.,** Receptor-mediated control of cholesterol metabolism, *Science,* 191, 150, 1976.
83. **Hamilton, R. L.,** Synthesis and secretion of plasma lipoproteins, pharmacological control of lipid metabolism, *Adv. Exp. Med. Biol.,* 26, 7, 1972.
84. **Hamilton, R. L.,** Hepatic secretion and metabolism of high density lipoprotein, in *Disturbances in Lipid and Apoprotein Metabolism,* Dietschy, John N., Gotto, Antonio M., Jr., Ontko, Joseph A., Eds., Clinical Physiology Series, American Physiological Society, 1977, 155.
85. **Hamilton, R. L., Williams, M. C., Fielding, C. J., and Havel, R. J.,** Discoidal bilayer structure of nascent high density lipoproteins from perfused rat liver, *J. Clin. Invest.,* 58, 667, 1976.
86. **Forte, T., Norum, K. R., Glomset, J. A., and Nichols, A. V.,** Plasma lipoproteins in familial lecithin: cholesterol acyltransferase deficiency: structure of low and high density lipoproteins as revealed by electron microscopy, *J. Clin. Invest.,* 50, 1141, 1971.
87. **Felker, T., Fainaru, M., Hamilton, R. L., and Havel, R. J.,** Secretion of arginine rich apoprotein of rat serum, *J. Lipid Res.,* 18, 465, 1977.
88. **Windmueller, H. G., Herbert, P. N., and Levy, R. I.,** Biosynthesis of lymph and plasma lipoprotein apoprotein by isolated perfused rat liver and intestine, *J. Lipid Res.,* 14, 215, 1973.
89. **Glickman, R. M., Green, P. H. R., Lees, R. S., and Tall, A.,** Apoprotein A-I synthesis occurs in normal intestinal mucosa and in Tangier disease, *N. Engl. J. Med.,* 299, 1424, 1978.
90. **Schwartz, D. E., Liotta, L., Schaeffer, E. J., and Brewer, H. G., Jr.,** Localization of apoproteins A-I, A-II, and B in normal, Tangier, and abetalipoproteinemia intestinal mucosa, *Circulation 58* Suppl. II-op, 1978.
91. **Imaizumi, K., Fainaru, M., and Havel, R. J.,** Composition of proteins of mesentric lymph chylomicrons in the rat and alterations produced upon exposure of chylomicrons to blood serum and serum proteins, *J. Lipid Res.,* 19, 712, 1978.
92. **Havel, R. J., Kane, J. P., and Kashyap, M. L.,** Interchange of apolipoproteins between chylomicrons and high density lipoproteins during alimentary lipemia in man, *J. Clin. Invest.,* 52, 32, 1973.
93. **Roheim, P. S., Giez, L. I., and Eder, H. A.,** Extrahepatic synthesis of lipoproteins of plasma and chyle: role of the intestine, *J. Clin. Invest.,* 45, 297, 1966.
94. **Friedberg, S. and Reynolds, J. A.,** The molar ratio of the two major polypeptide components of human high density lipoprotein, *J. Biol. Chem.,* 251, 4005, 1976.
95. **Glangeaud, M. C., Eisenberg, S., and Olivecrona, T.,** Very low density lipoprotein: dissociation of apolipoprotein C during lipoprotein lipase induced lipolysis, *Biochim. Biophys. Acta.,* 486, 23, 1977.
96. **Anderson, D. W., Nichols, A. V., Pan, S. S., and Lindgren, F. T.,** High density lipoprotein distribution, *Atherosclerosis,* 29, 161, 1978.
97. **Mahley, R. W., Weisgraber, K. H., Annerarity, T. L., and Bersot, T. P.,** Identification of pro-arginine-rich apoprotein — a possible modulator of lipoprotein binding to cell surface receptors of human fibroblasts, *Circulation,* 56, 57, 1977.
98. **Kostner, G.,** Studies on the cofactor requirements for lecithin: cholesterol acyltransferase, *Scand. J. Clin. Lab. Invest.* 33: Suppl. 137, 1974.
99. **Fielding, C. J. and Fielding, P. E.,** Purification and substrate specificity of lecithin-cholesterol acyltransferase from human plasma *FEBS* 15, 355, 1971.
100. **Brown, W. V. and Bagnisky, M. L.,** Inhibition of lipoprotein lipase by an apoprotein of human very low density lipoprotein, *Biochem. Biophys. Res. Comm.,* 46, 375, 1972.
101. **Assman, G. and Brewer, H. B.,** Lipid-protein interactions in high density liporpoteins, *Proc. Natl. Acad. Sci. U.S.A.,* 71, 989, 1974.
102. **Eisenberg, S. and Rachmilewitz, D.,** Metabolism of rat plasma very low density lipoprotein. I. Fate in circulation of the whole lipoprotein, *Biochim. Biophys. Acta,* 326, 371, 1973.
103. **Shepherd, J., Packard, C. J., Gotto, A. M., Jr., and Taunton, O. D.,** A comparison of two methods to investigate the metabolism of human apoproteins A-I and A-II, *J. Lipid Res.,* 19, 656, 1978.
104. **Cheung, M. C. and Albers, J. J.,** The measurement of apolipoprotein A-I and A-II levels in men and women by innumoassay, *J. Clin. Invest.,* 60, 43, 1977.
105. **Lux, S. E., Levy, R. I., Gotto, A. M., and Fredrickson, D. S.,** Studies on the protein defect in Tangier disease, isolation, and characterization of an abnormal high density lipoprotein, *J. Clin. Invest.,* 51, 2505, 1972.
106. **Goldstein, J. L. and Brown, M. S.,** Lipoprotein receptors, cholesterol metabolism, and atherosclerosis, *Arch. Pathol.,* 99, 181, 1975.
107. **Kayden, H. J., Hatam, L., and Beratis, N. G.,** Regulation of 3-hydroxy-3-methylglutanyl coenzyme A reductase activity and the esterification of cholesterol in human long term lymphoid cell lives, *Biochem.,* 15, 521, 1976.
108. **Blodavsky, I., Fielding, P. E., Fielding, C. J., and Gospodarowicz, D.,** Role of contact inhibition in the regulation of receptor-mediated uptake of low density lipoprotein in cultured vascular endothelial cells, *Proc. Natl. Acad. Sci., U.S.A.,* 75, 356, 1978.

109. **Angel, A., D'Costa, M. A., and Yuen, R.,** Low density lipoprotein binding internalization and degradation in human adipose cells, *Can. J. Biochem.*, 57, 578, 1979.
110. **Fogelman, A. M., Edmond, J., Polito, A., and Popjak, G.,** Control of lipid metabolism in human leukocytes, *J. Biol. Chem.*, 248, 6928, 1973.
111. **Avigan, J., Steinberg, D., and Berman, M.,** Distribution of labeled cholesterol in animal tissues, *J. Lipid Res.*, 3, 216, 1962.
112. **Field, H. Jr., Swell, L., Schools, P. E., and Treadwell, C. R.,** Dynamic aspects of cholesterol metabolism in different areas of the aorta and other tissues in man and their relationship to atherosclerosis, *Circulation*, 22, 547, 1960.
113. **Goodman, D. S.,** Cholesteryl ester metabolism, *Physiol. Rev.*, 45, 747, 1965.
114. **Farkas, J., Angel, A., and Avigan, M. I.,** Studies on the compartmentation of lipids in adipose cells. II. Cholesterol accumulation and distribution in adipose tissue components, *J. Lipid Res.*, 14, 344, 1973.
115. **Hirsch, E. G. and Han, P. W.,** Cellularity of rat adipose tissue: effects of growth, starvation and obesity, *J. Lipid Res.*, 10, 77, 1969.
116. **Glomset, J.,** The plasma lecithin:cholesterol acyltransferase reaction, *J. Lipid Res.*, 9, 155, 1968.
117. **Fredrickson, D. S., Gotto, A. M., and Levy, R. I.,** Familial lipoprotein deficiency, in *Metabolis Basis of Inherited Disease*, Stanbury, J. B., Wyngaarden, J. B., and Fredrickson, D. S., Eds., McGraw-Hill, New York, p. 493, 1972.
118. **Miller, G. J. and Miller, N. E.,** Plasma high density lipoprotein concentration and development of Ischaemic Heart Disease, *Lancet*, 1, 16, 1975.
119. **Miller, N. E., Nestel, P. J., and Clifton-Bligh, P.,** Relationships between plasma lipoprotein cholesterol concentration and the pool size and metabolism of cholesterol in man, *Atherosclerosis*, 23, 535, 1976.
120. **Stein, Y. and Stein, O.,** Cholesterol removal in isolated cells and in tissue culture, *Triangle*, 15, 63, 1976.
121. **Miller, N. E., Rao, S., Lewis, B., Bjorsvik, G., Myher, K., and Mjos, O. D.,** High density lipoprotein and physical activity, *Lancet*, 1,111, 1979.
122. **Carew, T. E., Koschinsky, T., Hayes, S. B., and Steinberg, D.,** A mechanism by which high density lipoproteins may slow the atherogenic process, *Lancet*, 2, 1315, 1976.
123. **Bjorkhem, I. and Lewenhaupt, A.,** Preferential utilization of newly synthesized cholesterol as substrate for bile acid biosynthesis, *J. Biol. Chem.*, 254, 5252, 1979.
124. **Bjorkhem, I. and Danielsson, H.,** 7a-Hydroxylation of exogenous and endogenous cholesterol in rat liver microsomes, *Eur. J. Biochem.*, 53, 63, 1975.
125. **Schwartz, C. C., Halloran, L. G., Vlahcevic, Z. R., Gregory, D. H., and Swell, L.,** Preferential utilization of free cholesterol from high-density lipoproteins in biliary cholesterol secretion in man, *Science*, 200, 62, 1978.
126. **Schwartz, C. C., Berman, M., Vlahcevic, Z. R., Halloran, L. G., Gregory, D. H., and Swell, L.,** Multicompartmental analysis of cholesterol metabolism in man, Characterization of hepatic bile acid and biliary cholesterol precursor sites, *J. Clin. Invest.*, 61, 408, 1978.
127. **Gresham, G. A.,** Atherosclerosis, its causes and potential reversibility, *Triangle*, 15, 39, 1976.
128. **Bondjers, G. and Bjorkerud, S.,** Cholesterol transfer between arterial smooth muscle tissue and serum lipoproteins in vitro, *Artery*, 1, 3, 1974.
129. **Nichols, A. V. and Smith, L.,** Effect of very low-density lipoproteins on lipid transfer in incubated serum, *J. Lipid Res.*, 6, 206, 1965.
130. **Hashimoto, S., Dayton, S., and Alfin-Slater, R. D.,** Esterification of cholesterol by homogenates of atherosclerotic and normal aortas, *Life Sci.*, 12, 1, 1973.
131. **Proudlock, J. W. and Day, A. J.,** Cholesterol esterifying enzymes of atherosclerotic rabbit intima, *Biochim. Biophys. Acta*, 260, 716, 1972.
132. **Day, A. J. and Gould-Hurst, P. R. S.,** Cholesterol esterase activity of normal and atherosclerotic rabbit aorta, *Biochim. Biophys. Acta*, 116, 169, 1966.
133. **Howard, C. F. and Portman, O. W.,** Hydrolysis of cholesterol linoleate by a high speed supernatant preparation of rat and monkey aorta, *Biochim. Biophys. Acta*, 125, 623, 1966.
134. **Kothari, H. V., Bonner, M. J., and Miller, B. E.,** Studies on cholesterol ester hydroylyzing activity in lysosomes from normal human aortas, *Fed. Proc.*, 28, 447, 1969.
135. **Takano, T., Black, W., Peters, T. J., and DeDube, C.,** Assay, kinetics, and lysosomal localization of an acid cholesterol esterase in rabbit aortic smooth muscle cells, *J. Biol. Chem.*, 249, 6732, 1974.
136. **Bailey, J. M.,** Lipid metabolism of cultured cells. IV. Serum alpha gobulins and cellular cholesterol exchange, *Exp. Cell Res.*, 37, 175, 1965.
137. **Werb, Z. and Cohn, A. A.,** Cholesterol metabolism in the macrophage. III. Ingestion and intracellular fate of cholesterol and cholesteryl esters, *J. Exp. Med.*, 135, 21, 1972.
138. **Hagerman, J. S. and Gould, R. G.,** The in vitro interchange of cholesterol between plasma and red cells, *Proc. Soc. Exp. Biol. Med.*, 78, 329, 1951.

139. **London, J. M. and Schwartz, H.**, Erythrocyte metabolism. The metabolic behavior of the cholesterol of human erythrocytes, *J. Clin. Invest.*, 32, 1248, 1953.

140. **Quarfordt, S. H. and Hildermans, H.**, Quantitation of the in vitro free cholesterol exchange of human red cells and lipoproteins, *J. Lipid Res.*, 11, 528, 1970.

141. **Bell, F. P. and Schwartz, C. J.**, Exchangeability of cholesterol between swine serum lipoproteins and erythrocytes, in vitro, *Biochim. Biophys. Acta*, 231, 553, 1971.

142. **Shinomiyo, M., Matsuoka, N., Shirai, K., Saito, Y., and Kumagai, A.**, Studies on cholesterol esterase in rat arterial wall, *Atherosclerosis*, 33, 343, 1979.

143. **Takano, T., Black, W. J., Peters, T. J., and DeDube, D.**, Assay, kinetics, and lysosomal localization of an acid cholesteryl esterase in rabbit aortic smooth muscle cells, *J. Biol. Chem.*, 249, 6732, 1974.

144. **Kothari, H. V., Miller, B. F., and Kritchevsky, D.**, Aortic cholesterol esterase — characteristics of normal rat and rabbit enzyme, *Biochim. Biophys. Acta*, 296, 446, 1973.

145. **Newman, H. A. K., Day, A. J., and Zilversmit, D. B.**, In vitro phospholipid synthesis in normal and atheromatous rabbit aortas, *Circ. Res.*, 19, 132, 1966.

146. **Vahouny, G. B., Weersing, S., and Treadwell, C. R.**, Function of specific bile acids in cholesterol esterase activity in vitro, *Biochim. Biophys. Acta*, 98, 607, 1965.

147. **Vahouny, G. V., Weersing, S., and Treadwell, C. R.**, Studies on an insoluble cholesterol-cholesterol esterase complex, *Arch. Biochem. Biophys.*, 112, 586, 1965.

148. **Behrman, H. R. and Armstrong, D. T.**, Cholesterol esterase stimulation by luteinizing hormone in luteinized rat ovaries, *Endocrinology*, 85, 474, 1969.

149. **Bonner, M. J., Miller, B. F., and Kothari, H. V.**, Lysosomal enzymes in aortas of species susceptible and resistant to atherosclerosis, *Proc. Soc. Exp. Biol. Med.*, 139, 1359, 1972.

150. **Brecher, P., Kessler, M., Clifford, C., and Chobanian, A.**, Cholesterol ester hydrolysis in aortic tissue, *Biochim. Biophys. Acta* 316, 386, 1973.

151. **Howard, C. F. and Portman, O. W.**, Hydrolysis of cholesteryl linoleate by a high speed supernatant preparation of rat and monkey aorta, *Biochim. Biophys. Acta*, 125, 623, 1966.

152. **Riddle, M. C., Fujimoto, W., and Ross, R.**, Two cholesterol ester hydrolases: Distribution in rat tissue and in cultured human fibroblasts and monkey arterial smooth muscle cells, *Biochim. Biophys. Acta*, 488, 359, 1977.

153. **Smith, E. B.**, The influence of age and atherosclerosis on the chemistry of aortic intima, Part 1 (The Lipids), *J. Atheroscler. Res.*, 5, 224, 1965.

154. **Sloan, H. R. and Fredrickson, D. S.**, Enzyme deficiency in cholesteryl ester storage disease, *J. Clin. Invest.*, 51, 1923, 1972.

155. **Eto, Y. and Suzuki, K.**, Cholesteol ester metabolism in the brain: properties and subcellular distribution of cholesterol-esterifying enzymes and cholesterol ester hydrolases in adult rat brain, *Biochim. Biophys. Acta*, 239, 293, 1971.

156. **Mueller, J. H.**, The mechanism of cholesterol absorption, *J. Biol. Chem.*, 27, 463, 1916.

157. **Nedswedski, S. W.**, Uber die Rolle der gallensauren salze beider fermentativen cholesterinestersynthese, Hoppe-Seyler's *Z. Physiol Chem.*, 239, 165, 1936.

158. **Klein, W.**, Uber die enzymatische hydrolyse der cholesterinester des menschlicen, Hoppe-Seyler's *Z. Physiol. Chem.*, 254, 1, 1938.

159. **Eto, Y. and Suzuki, K.**, Cholesterol ester metabolism in rat brain, *J. Biol. Chem.*, 248, 1986, 1973.

160. **Eto, Y. and Suzuki, K.**, Developmental changes of cholesterol ester hydrolases localized in myelin and microsomes of rat brain, *J. NeuroChem.*, 29, 1475, 1973.

161. **Hyun, J., Kothari, H., Hern, E., Mortenson, J., Treadwell, C. R., and Vahouny, G. V.**, Purification and properties of pancreatic juice cholesterol esterase, *J. Biol. Chem.*, 244, 1937, 1969.

162. **Proudlock, J. W. and Day, A. J.**, Cholesterol esterifying enzymes of atherosclerotic rabbit intima, *Biochim. Biophys. Acta*, 260, 716, 1972.

163. **Day, A. J. and Tume, R. K.**, Cholesterol-esterifying activity of cell-free preparations of rabbit peritoneal macrophages, *Biochim. Biophys. Acta*, 176, 367, 1969.

164. **Subbiah, M. T. R.**, Significance of various cholesterol ester hydrolases in aorta, *Steroids*, 33, 305, 1979.

Chapter 4

CHOLESTEROL CATABOLISM AND BILE ACID METABOLISM

Satindra Goswami and Jacqueline Dupont

TABLE OF CONTENTS

I. INTRODUCTION

The concentration of tissue cholesterol in mammals is ultimately controlled by the rate of its elimination from the metabolic pools. Cholesterol can be eliminated from the body through feces or urine or by epithelial sloughing and sebaceous secretions.[1] In humans, the loss of cholesterol by urinary elimination is negligible and the excretion of cholesterol from the skin is about 83 mg/day[2,3] which is quantitatively small compared to fecal loss.

Cholesterol can be excreted into feces in two major forms. One is as the neutral sterol and the other, the bile acid form. In the neutral sterol pathway, cholesterol enters the gastrointestinal lumen as a component of bile and mixes with dietary cholesterol and cholesterol derived from sloughing of intestinal mucosa and a gastrointestinal luminal cholesterol pool is established. This pool is subjected to reabsorption in the small intestine. The portion unabsorbed is metabolized by microflora in the large intestine and excreted in the feces.

For the bile acid form, cholesterol is transformed to bile acids in the liver and the bile acids are secreted as components of bile and become a part of the luminal pool in the intestine. Most of this pool is subject to reabsorption in the small intestine. The remainder is subjected to bacterial metabolism and excreted via the feces.

II. NEUTRAL STEROLS

A. Sources in the Gastrointestinal Tract

The fecal neutral sterols represent a mixture of derivatives of endogenous cholesterol and a varying amount of unabsorbed dietary sterols of animal and vegetable origin.[4] Cholesterol is the main sterol in foodstuffs of animal origin and β-sitosterol, campesterol, and stigmasterol comprise the main plant sterols.[5] In the intestinal lumen, biliary cholesterol is mixed with dietary cholesterol[6] and there is little difference between the two as precursors of neutral fecal sterols.[7] Among neutral sterols of endogenous origin, cholesterol, cholestanol, coprostanol, epicoprostanol, cholestanone, coprostanone, lathosterol, 7-dehydrocholesterol, and methosterol have been isolated from feces of various species.[5] Cholesteryl sulphate, has also been isolated from human feces[8] in the amount of about 5% of total fecal neutral sterols.[9] Some of the fecal neutral sterols mentioned are precursors of cholesterol and others are metabolites. In human feces, the precursors of cholesterol constitute a small percentage of total neutral sterols while in rats, the precursors might constitute a much higher percentage.[10]

B. Bacterial Transformations

During intestinal transit, cholesterol is mainly converted into two bacterial conversion products, coprostanol, and coprostanone. In their sterol balance studies using dietary β-sitosterol as a marker, Grundy et al.[11] noted that as much as 56% of neutral sterols were lost during their passage through the intestinal tract. They tentatively concluded that the losses were due to bacterial conversion of sterols to products which were no longer recognized as neutral sterols by the analytical methods used. A loss of up to 28% of added ^{14}C has been reported when feces from subjects fed a formula diet low in lactose and cellulose was incubated with 4-^{14}C cholesterol.[12] The loss was overcome by addition of cellulose and lactose to the man's diet. Cholesterol has been shown to be utilized as a sole source of carbon by a coliform organism isolated from man[13] and by mixed organisms isolated from rat feces.[14] Incubation of human and rat fecal homogenates with 4-^{14}C-cholesterol, however, did not produce $^{14}CO_2$ or other small relatively volatile fragments such as methane labeled with ^{14}C.[15,16] Thus, whatever might be the reason for these conflicting results, as long as the unidentified products (if any) have not been isolated and characterized, it will be generally accepted that the ring structure of cholesterol is not degraded in the mammalian system.

Cholesterol and plant sterols are transformed into a variety of different products by intestinal bacteria which makes the quantitative estimation of the neutral sterol fraction of feces a difficult task. Various methods[10,17-20] have been utilized for the quantitation of fecal neutral sterols, but the combined thin-layer chromatography-gas chromatography method of Miettinen et al.[10] takes advantage of the separation of neutral sterols into cholesterol and plant sterol derivatives. This method does not require the use of radioisotopes in vivo and sterol balance in man, as well as in animals, can be studied. The daily rate of excretion of fecal neutral sterols in man and rat measured in several laboratories with a variety of methods have been summarized and compared with this method.[10]

The composition of the neutral sterol fraction of feces is influenced by diet and intestinal microflora. Wilson[21] has shown that rats fed 20% linoleic acid in a fat-free diet exhibited increased formation of coprostanol and increased excretion of neutral sterols, whereas palmitic acid at the same level had no influence on fecal sterol excretion. When polyunsaturated fats were substituted for saturated fats in the diet, an increase of fecal neutral sterol excretion has been observed.[22,25] Plant sterols significantly increase the fecal excretion of cholesterol and its neutral metabolites.[26] Various factors, such as cerebroside or cellulose content of the diet, germ free status, influence the excretion of neutral sterols.[27] Kellogg and Wostmann[28] have shown that the rate of excretion of fecal neutral sterols is somewhat faster in conventional than germ-free animals. This might be due to changes (a) in the physical properties of sterols by bacteria, and (b) in the intestinal transit time of cholesterol and its bacterial metabolites. Cholesterol elimination in the form of neutral sterols is equal to or greater than that of bile acids in man, whereas in rat, fecal excretion of cholesterol is relatively low compared to that of bile acids.[27]

III. BILE ACIDS

A. Formation from Cholesterol

Bloch et al.[29] showed the existence of a direct metabolic relationship between cholesterol and bile acids and Siperstein et al.[30] confirmed this observation by feeding labeled cholesterol to rats and finding the radioactivity mainly in the bile acid fraction of bile and feces. The quantitative importance of the bile acid pathway of cholesterol metabolism was first demonstrated by Friedman et al.[31] He found that at least 60% of the cholesterol injected into rats was converted and excreted as bile acids.

The bile acids in mammals are all hydroxyl derivatives of cholanic acids, a 24-carboxyl compound of the parent hydrocarbons, 5α- and 5β-cholane (Figure 1). The individual bile acids differ from each other in the number, positions, and stereo configurations of the hydroxyl groups which are designated as either the α- or the β-configuration. Allo-bile acids are derivatives of 5β-cholanic acids whereas others belong to 5α-cholanic acid derivatives. The trivial and systematic names and the nature of some of the bile acids in mammals are presented in Table 1.

Bile acids which are synthesized *de novo* in the liver are called primary bile acids, whereas secondary bile acids are formed from the metabolism of the primary bile acids by intestinal microorganisms. The two most abundant primary bile acids, cholic acid and chenodeoxycholic acid (chenic acid), are synthesized in the liver from cholesterol.[43] If one compares the formula of these two acids and that of cholesterol (Figure 1), it is apparent that the biosynthetic changes necessary to convert cholesterol to bile acids include:

1. Removal of carbons 25, 26, and 27 from the side chain and conversion of carbon 24 to a carboxyl group.

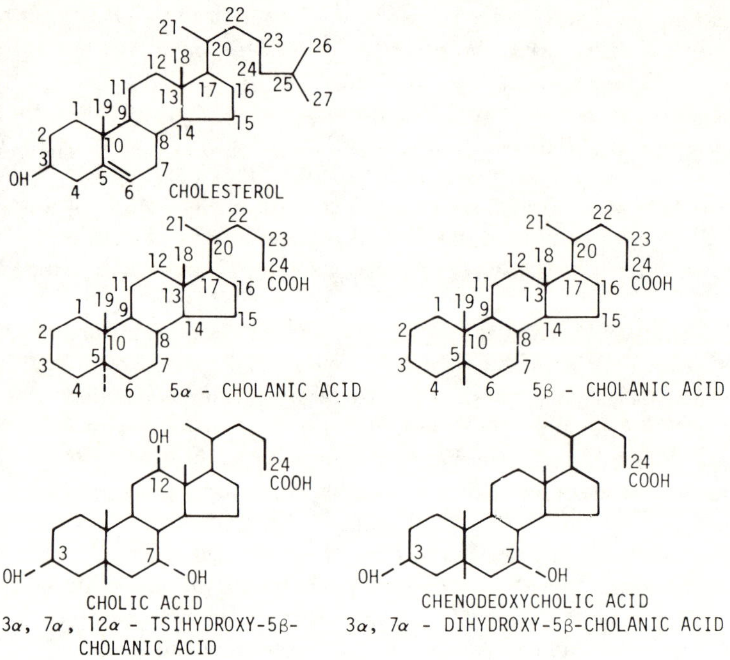

CHOLESTEROL

5α - CHOLANIC ACID

5β - CHOLANIC ACID

CHOLIC ACID
3α, 7α, 12α - TSIHYDROXY-5β-CHOLANIC ACID

CHENODEOXYCHOLIC ACID
3α, 7α - DIHYDROXY-5β-CHOLANIC ACID

FIGURE 1. Structural formulas of cholesterol, cholanic acids, and two commonly occurring primary bile acids.

2. Inversion of the hydroxyl group at position 3 from β to α configuration.
3. Insertion of hydroxyl groups on the steroid nucleus on carbon 7 or on carbons 7 and 12.
4. Saturation of the double bond between carbons 5 and 6.

The biosynthesis of primary bile acids from cholesterol has been extensively reviewed.[50-54] Bile acids formed in the liver are conjugated at position 24 (Figure 1) with either glycine or taurine before being secreted into the bile.[55] These conjugation reactions take place in liver microsomes.[56] Three α-sulphate esters of the commonly occurring bile acids have been shown to be present in rat and human bile.[57,58] The conjugated bile acids excreted with the bile enter into the gastrointestinal tract and most of them are rapidly reabsorbed. The reabsorbed bile acids return to the liver via the portal circulation where they are further metabolized and are resecreted into bile.

B. Bacterial Transformations

The bile acids found in the small intestine are mainly conjugated whereas in the cecum, they are found unconjugated.[59] Portman demonstrated that the splitting of the peptide bond occurs in the cecum.[60] Once the peptide bond is split, bile acids are transformed into a variety of products. The alteration of bile acids by the intestinal microflora include:

1. Bile acid deconjugation.
2. Dehydroxylation of bile acids at the carbon-7 position, e.g., from 3α, 7α to 3α; from 3α, 7α, 12α to 3α, 12α etc.
3. Dehydroxylation at the carbon-7 position together with oxidation at carbon-3 and carbon-12 positions, e.g., from 3α, 7α to 3-Keto, from 3α, 7α, 12α to 3α, 12-Keto and 3, 12-Diketo, etc.

Table 1
OCCURRENCE OF BILE ACIDS IN SOME MAMMALS

Species	Systematic name	Primary bile acids (trivial name)	Secondary bile acids (trivial name)	Nature of conjugation	Fecal bile acids	Ref.
Man	3α,7α,12α-Trihydroxy-5β-cholanic acid 3α,7α-Dihydroxy-5β-cholanic acid 7α,12α-Dihydroxy-5β-cholanic acid 3α-Hydroxy-5β-cholanic acid	Cholic Ehenodeoxycholic	Deoxycholic Lithocholic	Glycine and taurine	Deoxycholic, lithocholic, 3β-Hydroxy cholanic, 12-Keto lithocholic, 7-Keto deoxycholic, 3β, 12α-Dihydroxy-5β-cholanic, 7-Keto lithocholic acid, etc.	32-34
Rat	3α,6β,7α-Trihydroxy-5β-cholanic acid 3α,6β,7β-Trihydroxy-5β-cholanic acid 3α,7β-Dihydroxy-5β-cholanic acid	Cholic, chenodeoxycholic, α-Muricholic, β-Muricholic Ursodeoxycholic	Deoxycholic, lithocholic 7-Ketodeoxycholic, 12-Keto-lithocholic	Glycine and taurine	Deoxycholic, 12-Keto lithocholic, 7-Keto-5β-cholanic, Lithocholic, 3α,7β,12α-Trihydroxy cholanic acid, etc.	34-40
Pig	3α,6α,7α-Trihydroxy-5β-cholanic 3α,6α-Dihydroxy-5β-cholanic acid	Chenodeoxycholic Hyocholic	Lithocholic Hydeoxycholic	Taurine and glycine		41-44
Rabbit	3β-Hydroxy-5β-Cholanic acid 3α-12α-Dihydroxy-5α-cholanic acid	Chenodeoxycholic Cholic	Lithocholic Deoxycholic	Glycine	Deoxycholic, 3β-Hydroxycholanic 12-Keto lithocholic, 3, 12- Diketo-cholanic, 3β, 12α-Di-hydroxy cholanic Isolitho cholic, Allodeoxycholic, 12-Keto isolitholic, 3α,12α-Dihydroxy-5β-cholanic acid, etc.	34, 45-47

Table 1 (continued)
OCCURRENCE OF BILE ACIDS IN SOME MAMMALS

Mouse	3α-,6α,7β-Trihydroxy-5β-cholanic acid	Cholic, cheno-Deoxycholic, α-Muricholic, β-Muricholic	Deoxycholic, Lithocholic, ω-Muricholic	Taurine	Deoxycholic, lithocholic ω-Muricholic, cholic acid-7-sulfate, chenodeoxycholic acid-7-sulphate	48,49

4. Reduction of the resulting keto groups to both α- and β-hydroxyl groups, e.g., from 3α, 7-Keto to 3α, 7α and 3α, 7β etc.

The nature of the intestinal bacteria that metabolize the bile acids and the mechanisms of secondary bile acid formation in different species have been reviewed by Beher.[61] The metabolism of primary bile acids by intestinal microorganisms are depicted in Figure 2.

The fecal end products of bile acids are so varied in structure that their qualitative and quantitative assay pose a difficult task. Two types of methods are generally used for bile acid excretion studies. One is the isotope method[62-64] and the other is the chemical method.[65,66] A comparison of the two methods has also been made.[67] A new method based upon recovery of ^3H_2O from 24,25 ^3H cholesterol has given results similar to the older methods.[68] The daily fecal excretion of bile acids in some species is shown in Table 2.

Since the metabolism of primary bile acids in the gastrointestinal tract is influenced by the intestinal microflora, it is reasonable to assume that changes in the bacterial population will affect bile acid excretion. When germ free rats are fed cholic acid, taurocholic acid is the only metabolite found in the feces[69] as opposed to conventional rats which contain a variety of free bile acids.[70] Bile acid excretion is less in germ free (9 mg/kg body wt/day) rats. Similar results of considerably less bile acid excretion have been found in germ free mice (29.3 mg/kg body wt/day as compared to 41.2 mg/kg body wt/day in conventional mice).[49]

C. Intestinal Metabolism of Bile Acids

1. Intestinal Absorption

Large quantities of bile salts are required and they are conserved by an efficient reabsorption process. Reabsorption is achieved by (a) active transport and (b) passive ionic and nonionic diffusion.[71] The active transport mechanism which is an energy requiring process facilitates rapid absorption of bile acid conjugates in the ileum.[72] Taurine conjugated and conjugated trihydroxy bile salts are transported more readily than glycine conjugated and conjugated dihydroxy bile salts, respectively.[73] Occurrence of mutual inhibition of transport by glycine and taurine conjugates has also been noted.[74] The kinetics of the active transport of a number of bile salts by rat ileal sacs has been determined.[75] In the human, the ileal transport system has different affinities for different bile acids.[76]

Passive absorption of bile salts is usually not a significant phenomenon quantitatively. In passive nonionic diffusion, the nonionized bile acids are absorbed, whereas in passive ionic diffusion completely ionized bile salts are absorbed by the gastrointestinal wall. At the normal ileal pH (pH 5.0 to 7.0), unconjugated bile salts (pK_as of 5 to 6.3) will be mostly nonionized, a significant amount of glycine-conjugated bile salts (pK_as of 4.3 to 5.2) will be nonionized whereas taurine-conjugated bile salts (pK_as of 1.8 to 1.9) will be almost entirely in the ionized form.[77] Since passive nonionic diffusion is much greater than the diffusion of charged particles,[78] free bile acids are absorbed more rapidly from extraileal sites than glycine conjugates, while the ionized taurine conjugates are almost totally dependent on the active transport site in the ileum for their absorption.[72] The effects of certain structural features of bile salts on the state of passive ionic diffusion in rat small intestine have been studied.[75] Absorption of bile acids by passive nonionic diffusion in the proximal small intestine have been shown in humans.[79] Passive bile salt absorption in the small intestine is normally a minor phenomenon but in certain pathological conditions, this type of absorption might predominate.

Bile salts are absorbed to a considerable extent from the colon probably by passive

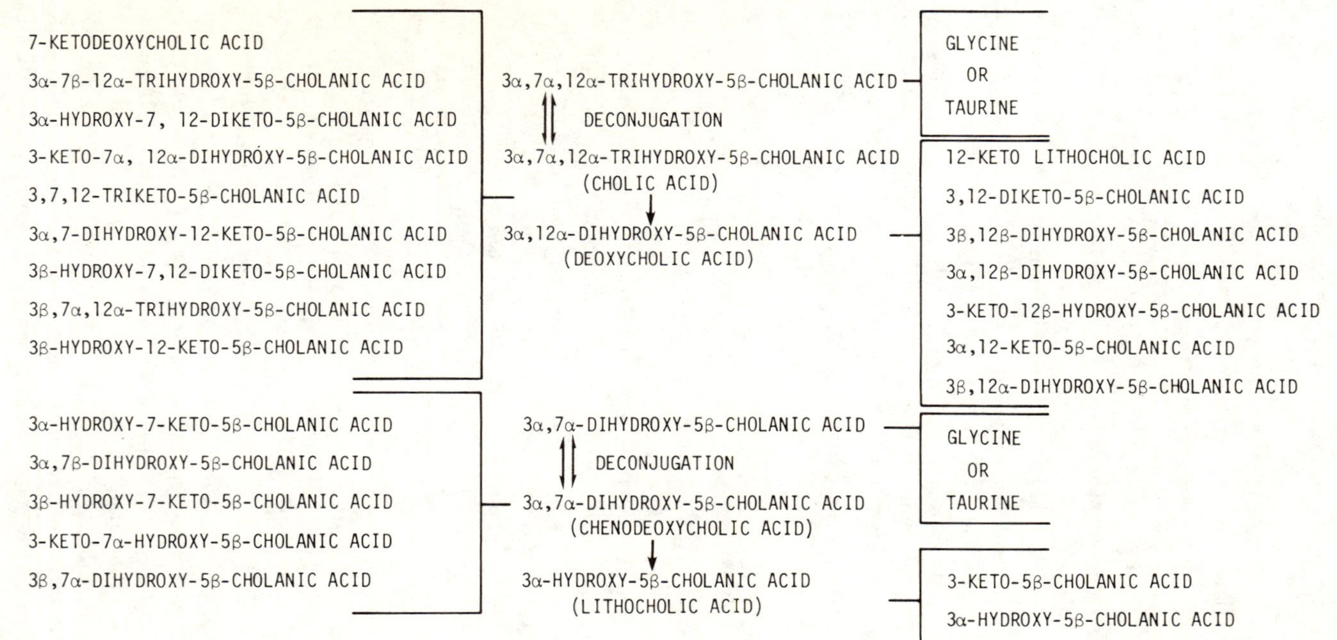

FIGURE 2. Metabolic products of two primary conjugated bile acids formed by the actions of intestinal microflora.

Table 2
DAILY FECAL EXCRETION OF BILE ACIDS REPORTED BY DIFFERENT LABORATORIES

Species	Method used	Daily fecal excretion of bile acid	Ref.
		mg/24 hr	
Man	Isotope	360	62
	Isotope	290	63
	Isotope	314±37	67
	Chemical	220-456	165
	Chemical	134-271	166
	Chemical	220±16	167
		mg/kg body wt/day	
Rat	Isotope	22	168
	Isotope	24	107
	Chemical	21.4	28
Rabbit	Isotope	27.5	169
	Chemical	24	170, 165
Mouse	Isotope	33.8	107
	Chemical	41.2	49

ionic and nonionic diffusion and the colonic absorption of secondary bile salts by humans has been calculated to be about 200 mg/day.[80] Studies have revealed that in man about 80% of bile acids are normally absorbed in the conjugated form and 20% as free acids. Reabsorption of both dihydroxy bile acids, e.g., deoxycholic and chenic acid, in man appear to be similar to and perhaps even better than that of cholic acid.[81] Bile salts have also been shown to be absorbed by damaged gall bladder mucosa.[82]

In summary, it can be concluded that bile salt absorption takes place at all levels of the gastrointestinal tract. Taurine-conjugates are absorbed in the lower ileum by both active transport and passive ionic diffusion, and glycine-conjugates are absorbed in the jejunum by passive ionic diffusion while absorption of free bile acids appears to take place by both active and passive ionic and nonionic diffusion. For further details, reviews by Wiener and Lack,[72] Dietschy[71] and Lack and Weiner[83] may be consulted.

The quantitation of the reabsorption of bile acids is difficult in man. It is generally calculated as the difference between the daily rate of biliary secretion and the daily fecal excretion which equals synthesis or turnover determined by isotope dilution techniques. The capacity of the intestine to reabsorb bile acids is not known but an estimation of 5 to 33 g/day has been made.[84] A marked increase in reabsorption might take place in obesity.[85] Under normal conditions, about 95% of the bile acids are absorbed and the rest are excreted via the feces.

2. *Intestinal Secretion*

The secretion of bile salts from the liver has been characterized as a saturable process and the secretory transport maxima of bile acids have been determined in some species.[86,87] Apparently a common transport process is shared by the major bile acids with differing affinities, causing competitive inhibition for excretion.[88] The secretion and metabolism of bile salts depend upon their hepatic uptake from the portal blood. The peripheral venous blood and the portal blood mix in the liver and as liver efficiently removes bile salts from the portal circulation, very little bile acids are present in peripheral blood in the normal state, e.g., 2 to 3.48 μmol/ℓ in man[89,90] and 80 μg/100 mℓ in the rat.[91] The bile acid concentrations, on the other hand, are much higher in the portal blood, e.g., 22.16 μmol/ℓ in man[90] and 66 to 237 μg/100 mℓ in rats.[92]

The kinetics and the mechanisms of bile salt uptake by the liver have been studied recently. Studies of the uptake of taurocholate in the dog[93,94] and in the rat[95,96] have shown that it is a saturable process. Taurochenodeoxycholate uptake is lower than that of taurcholate in the dog liver.[94] In man, the hepatic uptake of cholic acid is about 90%, whereas, that of chenic and deoxycholic acids is about 70%.[90] The conjugated trihydroxy bile acids and the conjugated monohydroxy bile acids are cleared more rapidly from circulation than the conjugated dihydroxy and the unconjugated bile acids respectively.[97] Differences in hepatic uptake of bile acids may be related to some extent to the binding of bile acids to proteins, e.g., dihydroxy bile acids, conjugated or unconjugated, were bound to albumin more tightly than trihydroxy conjugates,[97,98] and uptake is proportional to the availability of nonbound bile acid. It has been speculated, however, that intestinal absorption rather than protein binding could explain the observed differences.[90,97]

3. Enterohepatic Circulation

Bile is produced continuously by the liver but in most animals, it is required in the intestine only periodically. Conjugated bile acids synthesized in the liver are the main components in bile. The bile salts exert their function in the intestine only intermittently, i.e., during digestion when they participate in lipid absorption. These conflicting requirements of continuous secretion and periodic delivery in most vertebrates are reconciled by storing bile, between meals, in the gall bladder. During its stay in the gall bladder, the bile is concentrated and its composition is altered. When food enters the duodenum, cholecystokinin-pancreozymin (a hormone, secreted by the duodenum) is released; this facilitates the contraction and emptying of the gall bladder and the bile, containing bile salts, enters the lumen of the small intestine via the common bile duct. The absence of a gall bladder in a few mammals, like rat and horse, means the bile passes directly from the liver to the small intestine.

Following absorption, bile acids, free or conjugated, are transported to the liver via portal blood bound to albumin[99] and are cleared from the portal circulation.[100] The transported bile acids are mixed with newly synthesized bile acids in the liver, conjugated with taurine and/or glycine and once again secreted as a component of bile. This whole process of recycling is called the enterohepatic circulation and the amount of bile acids participating in this recirculation is called the bile acid pool size.

4. The Bile Acid Pool

Lindstedt[101] introduced the descriptive concept of bile acid kinetic pool. The principle of the method of measurement is based upon the assumption that the total bile acid pool is contained in the enterohepatic system. A radiotracer dose of cholic acid would, therefore, come into equilibrium with all the cholic acid in the system and its dilution over time would represent replacement by newly synthesized cholic acid. Extrapolation of the disappearance curve to zero time would provide an estimate of dilution of the tracer by the total pool and allow computation of the pool size. This technique has been used with variations in man and laboratory animals.[102,103] Another method of determining pool size is termed "the washout method".[104] This process requires a bile fistula and draining out of all the bile salts in the EHC.

Most of the mass of the bile acid pool is located in the small intestine (97%),[105] and the rest in the liver. The amount of the pool excreted per day is only 1 to 5% of the total,[106] and this amount is equated to rate of synthesis in the steady state. The number of enterohepatic cycles/day and the percent reabsorption would determine the net flux of bile acids and the amounts excreted and replaced by synthesis.

The pool size varies from species to species.[107] In humans it is about 3 gm.[108] White men have been reported to have a larger pool (2.91 gm) than women (2.34 gm).[109]

The determination of the number of cycles of enterohepatic circulation in man is a difficult task. It is generally measured by dividing the daily biliary secretion rate by the pool size. It has been calculated that the bile acid pool circulates 3 to 14 times daily in healthy man and this recycling may depend upon calorie intake.[110] Cycling results in secretion of 13 to 45 gm/day.[6]

Cycling frequency is greater in meal eating than fasting, but does not cease even in fasting.[106] The total secretion appears to adjust to a constant amount per day whether food is available continuously or intermitently.[106] Altering transit time in the intestine appears to cause a reciprocal alteration in secretion rate, with a net effect of keeping the bile acid pool size constant.[111]

Bile acid pool size and relative concentrations of cholesterol, bile acids and phospholipids are of importance in relation to cholesterol gallstone formation[112] and other disturbances of enterohepatic circulation.[113] The cholesterol saturation of bile (lithogenic index) is determined by its ratio to bile salts and lecithin. Lithogenicity of bile may be calculated if the total and relative lipid concentrations are known.[114]

If liver rapidly removes the circulating bile acids, then serum bile acids should reflect intestinal absorption. Acute or chronic interruption of the enterohepatic circulation has been shown to decrease the serum bile acid level,[115] whereas eating raises it. Conjugated chenic acid in serum rises after eating and stays at that level for several hours while conjugated cholic acid does not rise for about an hour and the level then falls off half an hour later.[116] This postprandial elevation of bile acids has been considered to represent incomplete hepatic clearance. It appears that in healthy subjects one maintains a level of serum bile acids only because of continuous absorption from the intestine and the elevations of bile acids in peripheral blood during digestion reflect a spillover during the constant hepatic clearance of the excess bile acids absorbed by the intestine.[117]

Factors which might affect the enterohepatic circulation are not clearly understood. This process is reduced by:

1. Damaged intestinal mucosa, either by inflammation or atrophy
2. Decreased absorptive surface, as in ileal exclusion
3. Decreased intestinal motility resulting in improper mixing of the intestinal contents
4. Binding of bile acids to some components of intestinal contents, e.g., cholestyramine, dietary fiber, bacteria, etc.
5. Alteration of the chemical structure of bile acids by bacteria.[85]

The interruption of the enterohepatic circulation with concomitant malabsorption of bile acids has been associated with bile acid diarrhea,[118] fatty acid diarrhea,[118] and enteric hyperoxaluria.[119]

D. Functions of Bile Acids

The functions of bile salts in the digestive tract have been summarized by Borgstrom[120] as follows:

1. The general detergent function of dispersing and solubilizing dietary fats and their hydrolytic products in micellar form facilitating their uptake into the intestinal cell membrane. In the absence of bile salts, the absorption of dietary fat and fat soluble vitamins will be impaired and cholesterol absorption will be entirely absent.
2. Effects on the functions of pancreatic lipolytic enzymes, e.g., an interaction with pancreatic lipase-colipase, sterol ester hydrolase, and dispersion of water insoluble long chain phosphoglycerides in the mixed micellar state which serves as substrate for phospholipase A_2.

3. Stimulation of the secretion of water and salt from the small and large intestine.
4. Effect on the motility of the intestine and the secretion of intestinal hormones. The intestinal microflora, by transforming some of the metabolic products of primary bile acids and thus removing them from the enterohepatic circulation, or by changing the motility of the gastrointestinal tract, influence bile acid excretion rates.

1. Absorption of Dietary Fat

The process of absorption of fat by the small intestine illustrates the unique functions of lipids in animal life. The insolubility of lipids in water necessitates a series of physical and metabolic events which are characteristic of lipid transport processes in numerous metabolic systems. Physical mixing of food occurs in the mouth and stomach and digestion of lipid begins the small intestine. Actions of lipase, colipase, calcium, and bile salts are required. Bile salts have several functions in the processes.[121]

Lipases act upon water insoluble substrates. In the intestine, the lipid is present in emulsified form; aggregates of lipid dispersed in an aqueous medium. Pancreatic lipase secreted into the intestine via the common bile duct binds to the surface of the emulsion droplet. This process is inhibited by bile salts which also bind to the oil droplet, displacing lipase. The relative concentrations of lipase and bile salts in the intestine result in the ability of the bile salts to totally inhibit the action of lipase. A small protein, colipase, (10,000 D) also secreted by the pancreas, reverses the effect of bile salts.[122] Colipase has a binding site for fat droplets[123] and for lipase, enabling lipase to come into contact with the triglycerides of the oil droplet. The sequence of events following has been observed visually by light microscopy.[124] The action of lipase in the presence of colipase and bile salts resulted in formation of a liquid crystalline phase, followed by extrusion of unhydrolyzed oil to form a separate oil droplet with the product protonated fatty acids and monoglycerides located in a "viscous isotropic" phase as described by Patton and Carey.[124] Without bile salts, extrusion of the unhydrolyzed oil droplet did not occur.

The viscous isotropic aggregate appears to be dispersed to a mixed micellar phase requiring the presence of bile acids. The bile originally secreted to the intestine was in the form of a mixed micelle with lecithin and cholesterol. Bile acid concentration must be high enough for ensuring micellar structure, i.e., there is a "critical micellar concentration" which must be maintained or the fatty acids and cholesterol will become insoluble and reform emulsion droplets. The ratio of bile salt to fatty acid must be 2 to 4 to attain clear micellar solutions.[121] The micelle solubilizes the cholesterol and fat soluble vitamins present in the gut lumen.

The critical function of the micelle is to bring the lipids through the unstirred water layer to the mucosal cells.[122] Micellar solubilization increases the aqueous concentration of lipolytic products 100 to 1000 times, thereby increasing the diffusion flux through the unstirred layer by 100 to 200 times. The functin of bile acids in fatty acid digestion is completed at this stage. Cholesterol absorption requires additional participation of bile acids.

2. Absorption of Cholesterol

The transport of cholesterol from the lumen of the small intestine to the lymph takes place via three steps:[125] transfer from lumen into the intestinal mucosa; metabolic changes in the mucosa; transport into lymph.

Cholesterol from dietary and endogenous sources is mixed with other secretory products of the gastrointestinal tract in the lumen of the small intestine. Cholesteryl esters, if present, are hydrolyzed by pancreatic sterol ester hydrolase in the presence of bile acids to free cholesterol and fatty acids. The process is presumed to be analogous to

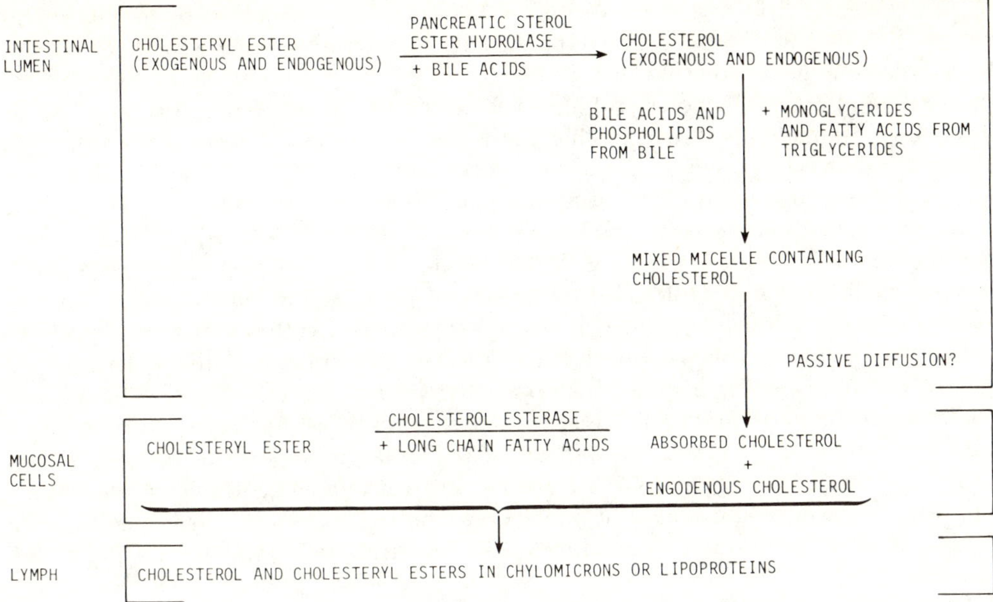

FIGURE 3. Schematic representation of cholesterol absorption process.

that for lipase-colipase.[123] The free cholesterol in the micelle is taken up by the mucosal cell presumably by passive diffusion. A major portion, about 70 to 90%, is reesterified to cholesteryl esters before incorporation into chylomicrons. The process is illustrated in Figure 3. In the absence of both bile and pancreatic juice, cholesterol esterifying activity essentially disappears from the intestinal mucosa.[125] Recent evidence indicates that pancreatic sterol ester hydrolase is essential in mucosal esterification of absorbed cholesterol. The pancreatic cholesterol esterase system requires trihydroxy bile salts as cofactors in the synthesis or hydrolysis of cholesteryl oleate, and this cofactor requirement is not related to the detergent properties of the bile salt.[12] The authors reported that cholic acid protects cholesterol esterase against proteolyic inactivation. Based on these findings they postulated that (1) bile salt complexed to the allosteric enzyme at or near the active site, or (2) produced a configurational change in the protein. They also reported formation of insoluble sterol-enzyme complexes using various sources of cholesterol esterase.

Cholesterol thus absorbed is carried via the thoracic duct to the systemic circulation and 90 to 95% of the chylomicron cholesterol is rapidly taken up by the liver.[127] (See Chapter 3.) Absorption of cholesterol by the gall bladder has been demonstrated recently.[128]

E. Regulation of Bile Acid Metabolism

Investigation of regulation of bile acid synthesis was initiated by studies of feedback inhibition by oral or infused bile acids.[129] These studies, using selected radioactive substrates as possible intermediates led to demonstration of the sequence of enzymic actions from cholesterol to primary bile acids.[130] The controlling role of cholesterol 7α-hydroxylase as the first and rate limiting step has been reviewed.[131] The microsomal enzyme requires cytochrome P_{450} NADPH, O_2,[131] and succinate as a respiratory substrate.[132] Microsomal enzymes complete the synthetic process including conjugation with glycine or taurine.[132]

One of the major aspects of regulation of formation of bile acids is the access of cholesterol to 7α-hydroxylase. Not all the liver or microsomal cholesterol is accessible to the enzyme.[133] The enzyme does not appear to be saturable by physiological means.[134] A number of studies have been made to determine the origin of the cholesterol accessible to 7α-hydroxylase. Endogenous vs. exogenous,[133] and newly synthesized vs. equilibrated[135] cholesterol have been examined as preferred substrates. All of these have been shown to be possible substrates. In the intact rat newly synthesized cholesterol has been shown to contribute 25% of the bile acid precursor, while equilibrated cholesterol made up 75% of newly synthesized bile acid.[136] In man, 31% of the bile acid precursor cholesterol was estimated to be newly synthesized in a study where bile fistulation prevented recycling.[137] The mode of identification of cholesterol for compartmentalization for bile acid synthesis is yet to be determined.

Formation of bile acids follows a diurnal rhythm.[131] Synthesis of the enzyme 7α-hydroxylase appears to be the mechanism for the variation in activity.[138] The diurnal cycle is not abolished by fasting,[131] adrenalectomy, or ocular enucleation.[139] Feedback inhibition of bile acid synthesis by enterohepatic circulation has been discussed in relation to regulation of bile acid pool size. The regulation appears to be mediated by 7α-hydroxylase.[131] Interruption of EHC results in accelerated synthesis of bile acids[140] and restoration or enhancement of bile acid flux inhibits synthesis.[129] The mechanism of the effect is not known. The nature of the bile acids influences the regulating enzymes.[141]

Diet influences the excretion of bile acids. Dietary cellulose,[142] pectin,[143] lignin[144] soybean meal[145] have been shown to increase bile acid excretion rates. Dietary studies with saturated and unsaturated fats in rats are confusing and the results are difficult to interpret. Some investigators have shown that dietary polyunsaturated fats increase the excretion of fecal bile acids[146,147] whereas others have found no significant effect on bile acid excretion when rats are fed diets containing either saturated or polyunsaturated fats.[148,149] In humans, the majority of the studies demonstrate an increased bile acid excretion with ingestion of polyunsaturated fats.[150,151]

The effects of carbohydrates,[152,85] vitamins,[153,154] hormones,[155,156] and drugs[157,158] on bile acid metabolism have also been studied. The results do not lend themselves to general interpretation.

Age and sex have some influence on bile acid metabolism. In the human fetus and newborn, most of the bile acids are conjugated with taurine and the glycine/taurine ratio reaches almost the adult level during the first year of life.[159,160] A small amount of ornithine conjugated cholic acid has also been found in newborns.[160] Excretion of cholesterol and bile acids has been reported to decrease with age in rats,[161,162] but others[163] have reported that only neutral sterol excretion decreased. On a whole animal basis, pool size, synthesis, secretion, and turnover frequency did not change with age.

Cholesterol fed female rats excrete significantly higher amounts of total bile acids and lithocholic acid in the feces than their male counterparts. No significant sex difference in the excretion of total bile acids has been noted in animals fed cholesterol-free diets although the amount of lithocholic acid excreted was significantly higher in the females.[164]

REFERENCES

1. **Chevallier, F.,** Dynamics of cholesterol in rats studied by the isotopic equilibrium method, *Adv. Lipid Res.*, Vol. 5, Paoletti, R. and Kritchevsky, D., Eds., Academic Press, New York, 1967, 209.
2. **Bhattacharya, A. K., Connor, W. E., and Spector, A. A.,** Excretion of sterols from the skin of normal and hypercholesterolemic humans. Implications for sterol balance studies, *J. Clin. Invest.*, 51, 2060, 1972.

3. **Nikkari, T., Schreibman, P. H., and Ahrens, E. H., Jr.**, In vivo studies of sterol and squalene secretion by human skin, *J. Lipid Res.*, 15, 563, 1974.
4. **Gould, R. G. and Cook, R. P.**, The metabolism of cholesterol and other sterols in the animal organism, in *Cholesterol, Chemistry, Biochemistry and Pathology*, Cook, R. P., Ed., Academic Press, New York, 1958, 237.
5. **Metzler, D. E.**, *Biochemistry. The chemical reactions of living cells*, Academic Press, New York, 1977, 731.
6. **Borgstrom, B.**, Studies on intestinal cholesterol absorption in the human, *J. Clin. Invest.*, 39, 809, 1960.
7. **Danielsson, H.**, Present status of research on catabolism and excretion of cholesterol, *Adv. Lipid Res.*, Vol. 1, Paoletti, R. and Kritchevsky, D., Eds., Academic Press, New York, 1963, 335.
8. **Moser, H. W., Moser, A. B., and Orr, J. C.**, Preliminary observations on the occurrence of cholesterol sulfate in man, *Biochem. Biophys. Acta*, 116, 146, 1966.
9. **Eneroth, P. and Hystrom, E.**, Quantification of cholesteryl sulfate and neutral sterol derivatives in human feces after purification on lipophilic sephadex gels. Bile acids and steroids 188, *Steroids*, 11, 187, 1968.
10. **Miettinen, T. A., Ahrens, E. H., Jr., and Grundy, S. M.**, Quantitative isolation and gas-liquid chromatographic analysis of total dietary and fecal neutral steroids, *J. Lipid Res.*, 6, 411, 1965.
11. **Grundy, S. M., Ahrens, E. H., Jr., and Salen, G.**, Dietary β-sitosterol as an internal standard to correct for cholesterol losses in sterol balance studies, *J. Lipid Res.*, 9, 375, 1968.
12. **Denbesten, L., Connor, W. E., Kent, T. H., and Lin, D.**, Effect of cellulose in the diet on the recovery of dietary plant sterols from the feces, *J. Lipid Res.*, 11, 341, 1970.
13. **Curran, G. L. and Brewster, K. D.**, Cholesterol metabolizing *Escherichia* coli, preliminary report, *Bull. Johns Hopkins Hosp.*, 91, 58, 1952.
14. **Wainfan, E., Henkin, G., Rittenberg, S. C., and Marx, W.**, Metabolism of cholesterol by intestinal bacteria in vitro, *J. Biol. Chem.*, 207, 843, 1954.
15. **Wood, P. D. S. and Hatoff, D.**, Incubation of human fecal homogenates with 4-^{14}C-cholesterol, *Lipids*, 5, 720, 1969.
16. **Levitt, M. D., Hanson, R. F., Bond, J. H., and Engel, R. R.**, Failure to demonstrate degradation of (4-^{14}C) cholesterol to volatile hydrocarbons in rats and in human fecal homogenates, *Lipids*, 10, 662, 1975.
17. **Wilson, J. D.**, The quantification of cholesterol excretion and degradation in the isotopic steady state in the rat: the influence of dietary cholesterol, *J. Lipid Res.*, 5, 409, 1964.
18. **Goldsmith, G. A., Hamilton, J. G., and Miller, O. N.**, Lowering of serum lipid concentrations: mechanisms used by unsaturated fats, nicotinic acid and neomysin excretion of sterols and bile acids, *Arch. Intern. Med.*, 105, 521, 1960.
19. **Bloomfield, D. K.**, Cholesterol metabolism. III. Enhancement of cholesterol absorption and accumulation in safflower oil-fed rats, *J. Lab. Clin. Med.*, 64, 613, 1964.
20. **Powell, R. C., Nunes, W. T., Harding, R. S., and Vacca, J. B.**, The influence of nonabsorbable antibiotics on serum lipids and the excretion of neutral sterols and bile acids, *Am. J. Clin. Nutr.*, 11, 156, 1962.
21. **Wilson, J. D.**, The effect of dietary fatty acids on coprostanol excretion by the rat, *J. Lipid Res.*, 2, 350, 1961.
22. **Nestel, P. J., Havenstein, N., Whyte, H. M., Scott, T. J., and Cook, L. J.**, Lowering of plasma cholesterol and enhanced sterol excretion with the consumption of polyunsaturated ruminant fats, *N. Eng. J. Med.*, 288, 279, 1973.
23. **Antonis, A. and Bersohn, I.**, The influence of diet on fecal lipids in South Africa white and Bantu prisoners, *Am. J. Clin. Nutr.*, 11, 142, 1962.
24. **Moore, R. B., Anderson, J. T., Taylor, H. I., Keys, A., and Frantz, I. D.**, Effect of dietary fat on the fecal excretion of cholesterol and its degradation products in man, *J. Clin. Invest.*, 47, 1517, 1968.
25. **Connor, W. E., Witiak, D. T., Stone, D. B., and Armstrong, M. L.**, Cholesterol balance and fecal neutral steroid and bile acid excretion in normal men fed dietary fats of different fatty acid composition, *J. Clin. Invest.*, 48, 1363, 1969.
26. **Kudchodkar, B. J., Horlick, L., and Sodhi, H. S.**, Effects of plant sterols on cholesterol metabolism in man, *Atherosclerosis*, 23, 239, 1976.
27. **Lutton, C.**, The role of the digestive tract in cholesterol metabolism, *Digestion*, 14, 342, 1976.
28. **Kellogg, T. F. and Wostmann, B. A.**, Fecal neutral steroids and bile acids from germfree rats, *J. Lipid Res.*, 10, 495, 1969.
29. **Bloch, K., Berg, B. N., and Rittenberg, D.**, The biological conversion of cholesterol to cholic acid, *J. Biol. Chem.*, 149, 511, 1943.
30. **Siperstein, M. D., Jayko, M. E., Chaikoff, J. L., and Dauben, W. G.**, Nature of the metabolism products of ^{14}C cholesterol excreted in bile and feces, *Proc. Soc. Exp. Biol. Med.*, 81, 720, 1952.

31. **Friedman, M., Byers, S. O., and Gunning, B.,** Observations concerning production and excretion of cholesterol in mammals. VIII. Fate of injected cholesterol in the animal body, *Am. J. Physiol.*, 172, 309, 1953.
32. **Eneroth, P., Gordon, B., Ryhage, R., and Sjovall, J.,** Identification of mono- and dihydroxy bile acids in human feces by gas-liquid chromatography and mass spectrometry, *J. Lipid Res.*, 7, 524, 1966.
33. **Eneroth, P., Gordon, B., and Sjovall, J.,** Characterization of trisubstituted cholanoic acids in human feces, *J. Lipid Res.*, 7, 524, 1966.
34. **Matschiner, J. T.,** Naturally occurring bile acids and alcohols and their origins, in *The Bile Acids, Chemistry, Physiology and Metabolism*, Vol. 1, Nair, P. P. and Kritchevsky, D., Eds., Plenum Press, New York, 1972, 11.
35. **Norman, A.,** On the conjugation of bile acids in the rat, *Acta Physiol. Scand.*, 32, 1, 1954.
36. **Lindstedt, S. and Norman, A.,** On the excretion of bile acid derivatives in feces of rats fed cholic acid-24-^{14}C and chenodeoxycholic acid-24-^{14}C, *Acta Physiol. Scand.*, 34, 1, 1955.
37. **Norman, A. and Sjoval, J.,** Microbial transformation products of cholic acid in the rat, *Biochim. Biophys. Acta*, 29, 467, 1958.
38. **Samuelsson, B.,** On the metabolism of ursodeoxycholic acid in the rat. Bile acids and steroids 84, *Acta Chem. Scand.*, 13, 970, 1959.
39. **Samuelsson, B.,** On the metabolism of chenodeoxycholic acid in the rat. Bile acids and steroids 85, *Acta Chem. Scand.*, 13, 976, 1959.
40. **Hsia, S. L., Elliott, W. H., Matschiner, J. T., Doisy, E. A., Jr., Thayer, S. A., and Doisy, E. A.,** Bile acids XIII. Further contributions to the constitution of muricholic acids, *J. Biol. Chem.*, 235, 1963, 1960.
41. **Haslewood, G. A. D.,** Comparative studies of "bile salts". 9. The isolation and chemistry of hyocholic acid, *Biochem. J.*, 62, 637, 1956.
42. **Haslewood, G. A. D. and Ogan, A. U.,** Taurine conjugates in pig bile salts, *Biochem. J.*, 67, 30p, 1957.
43. **Bergstrom, S., Danielsson, H., and Samuelsson, B.,** Formation and metabolism of bile acids, in *Lipid Metabolism*, Bloch, K., Ed., John Wiley & Sons, New York, 1960, 291.
44. **Haslewood, G. A. D.,** The biological significance of chemical differences in bile salts, *Biol. Rev.*, 39, 537, 1964.
45. **Hellstrom, K. and Sjovall, J.,** Metabolism of chenodeoxycholic acid in the rabbit. Bile acids and steroids, 104, *Acta Chem. Scand.*, 14, 1763, 1960.
46. **Danielsson, H., Kallner, A., and Sjovall, J.,** On the composition of the bile acid function of rabbit feces and the isolation of a new bile acid: 3α, 2α-dihydroxy-5α-cholanic acid, *J. Biol. Chem.*, 238, 3846, 1963.
47. **Taylor, W.,** The bile acid composition of rabbit and cat gall bladder bile, *J. Steroid Biochem.*, 8, 1077, 1977.
48. **Danielsson, H. and Kazuno, T.,** On the metabolism of bile acids in the mouse. Bile acids and steroids 84, *Acta Chem. Scand.*, 13, 1141, 1959.
49. **Eyssen, H. J., Parmentier, G. G., and Mertens, J. A.,** Sulfated bile acids in germ-free and conventional mice, *Eur. J. Biochem.*, 66, 507, 1976.
50. **Staple, E.,** Mechanism of cleavage of the cholestane side chain in bile acid formation, in *Bile Salt Metabolism*, Schiff, L., Carey, J. B., Jr., and Dietschy, J. M., Eds., Charles C Thomas, Springfield, 1969, 1927.
51. **Elliott, W. M. and Hyde, P. M.,** Pathways of bile acid synthesis, *Am. J. Med.*, 51, 568, 1971.
52. **Percy-Robb, I. W. and Boyd, G. S.,** The biosynthesis of bile acids, *Scot. Med. J.*, 18, 166, 1973.
53. **Mosbach, E. H. and Salen, G.,** Bile acid biosynthesis. Pathways and regulation, *Am. J. Dig. Dis.*, 19, 920, 1974.
54. **Danielsson, H. and Sjovall, J.,** Bile acid metabolism, *Ann. Rev. Biochem.*, 44, 233, 1975.
55. **Ekdahl, P. H. and Sjovall, J.,** On the conjugation and formation of bile acids in the human liver, *Acta Chem. Scand.*, 144, 439, 1957.
56. **Gardner, B. and Chenouda, M. S.,** Studies of bile acid secretion by isolated rat hepatocytes, *J. Lipid Res.*, 19, 985, 1978.
57. **Palmer, R. H.,** Bile acid sulfates. II. Formation, metabolism and excretion of lithocholic acid sulfates in the rat, *J. Lipid Res.*, 12, 680, 1971.
58. **Palmer, R. H. and Bolt, M. G.,** Bile acid sulfates. I. Synthesis of lithocholic acid sulfates and their identification in human bile, *J. Lipid Res.*, 12, 671, 1971.
59. **Norman, A. and Sjoval, J.,** On the transformation and enterohepatic circulation of cholic acid in the rat. Bile acids and steroids 68., *J. Biol. Chem.*, 233, 872, 1958.
60. **Portman, O. W.,** Further studies of the intestinal degradation products of cholic acid-24-^{14}C in rats. Formation of deoxycholic acid, *Arch. Biochem. Biophys.*, 78, 125, 1958.

61. **Beher, W. T.,** Bile Acids. Chemistry and physiology of bile acids and their influence of Atherosclerosis, in *Monographs on Atherosclerosis,* Vol. 6, Kritchevsky, D., Pollak, O. J., and Simms, H. S., Eds., S. Karger, Basel, 1976, 34.
62. **Lindstedt, S. and Norman, A.,** The turnover of bile acids in the rat, *Acta Physiol. Scand.,* 38, 121, 1956.
63. **Lindstedt, S.,** The turnover of cholic acid in man, *Acta Physiol. Scand.,* 40, 1, 1957.
64. **Rosenfeld, R. S. and Hellman, L.,** Excretion of steroid acids in man, *Arch. Biochem. Biophys.,* 97, 406, 1962.
65. **Grundy, S. M., Ahreans, E. H., Jr., and Miettinen, T. A.,** Quantitative isolation and gas-liquid chromatographic analysis of total fecal bile acids, *J. Lipid Res.,* 6, 397, 1965.
66. **Eneroth, P., Hellstrom, K., and Sjovall, J.,** A method for quantitative determination of bile acids in human feces, *Acta Chem. Scand.,* 22, 1729, 1968.
67. **Subbiah, M. T. R., Tyler, N. E., Buscaglia, M. D., and Marai, L.,** Estimation of bile acid excretion in man: comparison of isotopic turnover and fecal excretion methods, *J. Lipid Res.,* 17, 78, 1976.
68. **Rosenfeld, R. S., Bradlow, H. L., Levin, J., and Zumoff, B.** Preparation of {24,25-^{3}H} cholesterol. Oxidation in man as a measure of bile acid formation. *J. Lipid Res.,* 19, 850, 1978.
69. **Gustafsson, B. E., Bergstrom, S., Lindstedt, S., and Norman, A.,** Turnover and nature of fecal bile acids in germ free and infected rats fed cholic acid-24-^{14}C, *Proc. Soc. Expl. Biol. Med.,* 94, 467, 1957.
70. **Kellogg, T. F.,** Bile acid metabolism in gnotobiotic animals, in *The Bile Acids, Chemistry, Physiology and Metabolism,* Vol. 2, Nair, P. P. and Kritchevsky, D., Eds., Plenum Press, New York, 1973, 283.
71. **Dietschy, J. M.,** Mechanism for the intestinal absorption of bile salts, *J. Lipid Res.,* 9, 297, 1968.
72. **Weiner, I. M. and Lack, L.,** Bile salt absorption, enterohepatic circulation, *Handbook of Physiology,* Section 6, Vol. III, American Physiological Society, Washington, D.C., 1968, 1439.
73. **Lack, L. and Weiner, I. M.,** Intestinal bile salt transport structure-activity relationships and other properties, *Am. J. Physiol.,* 210, 1142, 1966.
74. **Heaton, K. W. and Lack, L.,** Ileal bile salt transport: mutual inhibition in an in vivo system, *Am. J. Physiol.,* 214, 585, 1968.
75. **Schiff, E. R., Small, N. C., and Dietschy, J. M.,** Characterization of the kinetics of the passive and active transport mechanisms for bile acid absorption in the small intestine and colon of the rat, *J. Clin. Invest.,* 51, 1351, 1972.
76. **Krag, E. and Phillips, S. F.,** Active and passive bile acid absorption in man. Perfusion studies of the ileum and jejunum, *J. Clin. Invest.,* 53, 1686, 1974.
77. **Dowling, R. H. and Small, D. M.,** The effect of pH on the solubility of varying mixtures of free and conjugated bile salts in solution, *Gastroenterology,* 54, 1291, 1968.
78. **Dietschy, J. M., Salomon, H. S., and Siperstein, M. D.,** Bile acid metabolism. I. Studies on the mechanisms of intestinal transport, *J. Clin. Invest.,* 45, 832, 1966.
79. **Angelin, B., Einarsson, K., and Hellstrom, K.,** Evidence for the absorption of bile acids in the proximal small intestine of normo- and hyperlipidaemic subjects, *Gut,* 17, 420, 1976.
80. **Samuel, P., Saypol, G. M., Meilman, E., Mosbach, E. H., and Chafizadeh, M.,** Absorption of bile acids from the large bowel in man, *J. Clin. Invest.,* 47, 2070, 1968.
81. **Hepner, G. W., Hofmann, A. F., and Thomas, P. J.,** Metabolism of steroid and amino acid moieties of conjugated bile acids in man. I. Cholyglycine, *J. Clin. Invest.,* 51, 1889, 1972.
82. **Ostrow, J. D.,** Absorption by the gall bladder of bile salts, sulfobromophthalein, and iodipamide, *J. Lab. Clin. Med.,* 74, 482, 1969.
83. **Lack, L. and Weiner, I. M.,** Bile salt transport systems, in *The Bile Acids,* Chemistry, physiology and metabolism, Vol. 2, Nair, P. P., and Kritchevsky, D., Eds., Plenum Press, New York, 1963, 33.
84. **Grundy, S. M. and Metzger, A. L.,** A physiological method for estimation of hepatic secretion of biliary lipids in man, *Gastroenterology,* 62, 1200, 1972.
85. **Miettinen, T. A.,** Bile acid metabolism, in *Handbook of Experimental Pharmacology,* Vol. 41, Kritchevsky, D., Ed., Springer Verlag, Berlin, 1975, 109.
86. **O'Maille, E. R. L., Richards, T. G. and Short, A. H.,** Conjugation of cholic acid and its uptake and secretion: hepatic extraction of taurocholate and cholate in the dog, *J. Physiol.,* 189, 337, 1967.
87. **Sperben, I.,** Biliary secretion of organic anions and its influence on bile flow, in *The Biliary System,* A symposium of the NATO advanced study institute, Taylor, W., Ed., Blackwell Scientific Oxford, 1965, 457.
88. **Sarfeh, I. J., Friday, S. E., and Balint, A.,** The dual effect of glycocholate on hepatic dihydroxy bile acid excretion, *J. Surg. Res.,* 25, 280, 1978.
89. **Pennington, C. R., Ross, P. E., and Bouchier, I. A. D.,** Fasting and postprandial serum bile acid concentrations in normal persons using an improved GLC method, *Digestion,* 14, 56, 1978.

90. **Ahlberg, J., Angelin, B., Bjorkem, I., and Einarsson, K.,** Individual bile acids in portal venous and systemic blood serum of fasting man, *Gastroenterology,* 73, 1377, 1977.
91. **Grundy, S. M. and Sjovall, J.,** Studies on bile acids in rat systemic blood, *Proc. Soc. Exp. Biol. Med.,* 107, 306, 1961.
92. **Barnes, S., Billing, B., and Morris, J. S.,** Effect of fasting and ileal resection on the concentration of deoxycholic acid in rat portal blood, *Proc. Soc. Exp. Biol. Med.,* 152, 292, 1976.
93. **Glasinovic, J. C., Dumont, M., Duval, M., and Erlinger, S.,** Hepatocellular uptake of taurocholate in the dog, *J. Clin. Invest.,* 55, 419, 1975.
94. **Hoffman, N. E., Donald, D. E., and Hofmann, A. F.,** Effect of primary bile acids on bile lipid secretion from perfused dog liver, *Am. J. Physiol.,* 229, 714, 1975.
95. **Reichen, J. and Paumgartner, G.,** Kinetics of taurocholate uptake by the perfused rat liver, *Gastroenterology,* 68, 132, 1975.
96. **Richen, J. and Paumgartner, G.,** Uptake of bile acids by perfused rat liver, *Am. J. Physiol.,* 231, 734, 1976.
97. **Cowen, A. E., Korman, M. G., Hofmann, A. F., and Thomas, P. J.,** Plasma disappearance of radioactivity after intravenous injection of labeled bile acids in man, *Gastroenterology,* 68, 1567, 1976.
98. **Rudman, D. and Kendall, F. E.,** Bile acid content of human serum. II. The binding of cholanic acids by human plasma proteins, *J. Clin. Invest.,* 36, 538, 1957.
99. **Burke, C. W., Lewis, B., Panveliwalla, D., and Tabaqchalia, S.,** The binding of cholic acid and its taurine conjugate to serum proeins, *Clin. Chim. Acta,* 32, 207, 1971.
100. **Tidball, C. S.,** Intestinal and hepatic transport of cholate and organic dyes, *Am. J. Physiol.,* 206, 239, 1974.
101. **Lindstedt, S. and Norman, A.,** The turnover of bile acids in the rat. Bile acids and steroids 39, *Acta Physiol Scand.,* 38, 121, 1957.
102. **Lindstedt, S.,** The turnover of cholic acid in man. Bile acids and steroids 51, *Acta Physiol Scand.,* 40, 9, 1957.
103. **Duane, W. C., Adler, R. D., Bennion, L. J., and Ginsberg, R. L.,** Determination of bile acid pool size in man: a simplified method with advantages of increased precision, shortened analysis time, and decreased isotope exposure, *J. Lipid Res.,* 16, 155, 1975.
104. **Mok, E. Y. I., Perry, P. M., and Dowling, R. H.,** The control of bile acid pool size: Effect of jejunal resection and phenobartitone on bile acid metabolism in the rat, *Gut,* 15, 247.
105. **Fisher, M. M., Kakis, G., and Yousef, I. M.,** Bile acid pool in Wistar rats, *Lipids,* 11, 93, 1976.
106. **Mok, H. Y. I., von Bergmann, K., and Grundy, S. M.,** Effects of continuous and intermittent feeding on biliary lipid outputs in man: application for measurements of intestinal absorption of cholesterol and bile acids, *J. Lipid Res.,* 20, 389, 1979.
107. **Beher, W. T., Filus, A. M., Rao, B., and Beher, M. E.,** A comparative study of bile acid metabolism in the rat, mouse, hamster and gerbil, *Proc. Soc. Exp Biol. Med.,* 130, 1067, 1969.
108. **Ponz de Leon, M., Ferenderes, R., and Carulli, N.,** Bile lipid composition and bile acid pool size in diabetes, *Dig Dis.,* 23, 710, 1978.
109. **Bennion, L. J., Dronbny, E., Knowler, W. C., Ginsberg, R. L., Garnick, M. B., Adler, R. D., and Duane, W. C.,** Sex differences in the size of bile acid pools, *Metabolism,* 27, 961, 1978.
110. **Brunner, H., Hofmann, A. F., and Summerskill, W. H. J.,** Daily secretion of bile acids and cholesterol measured in health, *Gastroenterology,* 62, 188, 1972.
111. **Hardison, W. G. M., Tomoaszewski, N., and Grundy, S. M.,** Effect of acute alterations in small bowel transit time upon the biliary excretion rate of bile acids, *Gastroenterology,* 76, 568, 1979.
112. **Bennion, L. J. and Grundy, S. M.,** Risk factors of the development of cholelithiasis in man, *N. Eng. J. Med.,* 299, 1161, 1978.
113. **Van Berge Henegouwen, G. P. and Hofmann, A. F.,** Clinical aspects of disturbances in the enterhepatic circulation of bile acids in man: the cholanopathies, *Neth. J. Med.,* 21, 257, 1978.
114. **Carey, M. C.,** Critical tables for calculating the cholesterol saturation of bile, *J. Lipid Res.,* 19, 945, 1978.
115. **LaRusso, N. F., Korman, M. G., Hoffman, N. E., and Hofmann, A. F.,** Intestinal absorption — the major determinant of serum bile acids in patients with normal liver function, *Gastroenterology,* 67, 806, 1974.
116. **LaRusso, N. F., Hoffman, N. E., Korman, M. G., Hofmann, A. F., and Cowen, A. E.,** Determinants of fasting and postprandial serum bile and acid levels in healthy man, *Am. J. Dig. Dis.,* 23, 385, 1978.
117. **Schalm, S. W., LaRusso, N. F., Korman, M. G., Cowen, A. E., Hoffman, N. E., Carter, J. A., Turcotte, J., and Hofmann, A. F.,** Diurnal variation of serum bile acids determined by multiple specific bile acid radioimmunoassays, *Clin. Res.,* 23, 396A, 1975.
118. **Hofmann, A. F.,** Bile acid malabsorption caused by ileal resection, *Arch. Intern. Med.,* 130, 597, 1972.

119. **Smith, L. H. and Hofmann, A. F.,** Acquired hyperoxaluria, urolithiasis and intestinal disease. A new digestive disorder? *Gastroenterology,* 66, 1257, 1974.
120. **Borgstrom, B.,** Bile salts — their physiological functions in the gastrointestinal tract, *Acta Med. Scand.,* 196, 1, 1974.
121. **Hofmann, A. F. and Mekhjian, H. S.,** Bile acids and the intestinal absorption of fat and electrolytes in health and disease, in *The Bile Acids,* Vol. 2, Nair, P. P. and Kritchevsky, D., Eds., Plenum Press, New York, 1973.
122. **Hofmann, A. F.,** Fat digestion: the interaction of lipid digestion products with micellar bile acid solutions, in *Lipid Absoroption: Biochemical and Clinical Aspects,* Rommel, D. and Bohmer, R., Eds., MTP Press, Lancaster, England, 1973, 3.
123. **Patton, J. S., Albertsson, P. A., Erlanson, C., and Borgstrom, B.,** Binding of porcine pancreatic lipase and colipase in the absence of substrate studied by two-phase partition and affinity chromatography, *J. Biol. Chem.,* 253, 4195, 1979.
124. **Patton, J. S. and Carey, M. C.,** Watching fat digestion, *Science,* 204, 145, 1979.
125. **Treadwell, C. R. and Vahouny, G. V.,** Cholesterol absorption, in *Handbook of Physiology,* Section 6, Vol. III, American Physiological Society, Washington, D.C., 1978, 1407.
126. **Gallo, L. L., Newbill, T., Hyun, J., Vahouny, G. V., and Treadwell, C. R.,** Role of pancreatic cholesterol esterase in the uptake and esterification of cholesterol by isolated intestinal cells, *Proc. Soc. Exp. Biol. Med.,* 156, 277, 1977.
127. **Goodman, D. S.,** Cholesterol ester metabolism, *Physiol. Rev.,* 45, 747, 1965.
128. **Neiderhiser, D. H., Harmon, C. K., and Roth, H. P.,** Absorption of cholesterol by the gall bladder, *J. Lipid Res.,* 17, 116, 1976.
129. **Shefer, S., Hauser, S., Bekersky, E., and Mosbach, E.,** Feedback regulation of bile acid biosynthesis in the rat, *J. Lipid Res.,* 10, 646, 1969.
130. **Mosbach, E. H. and Salen, G.,** Bile acid biosynthesis, pathways and regulation, *Dig. Dis.,* 19, 920, 1974.
131. **Myant, N. B. and Mitropoulos, K. A.,** Cholesterol 7α-hydroxylase, *J. Lipid Res.,* 18, 135, 1977.
132. **Gardner, B. and Chenouda, M. S.,** Studies of bile acid secretion by isolated rat hepatocytes, *J. Lipid Res.,* 19, 985, 1978.
133. **Balasubramaniam, S., Mitropoulos, K. A., and Myant, N. B.,** Evidence for the compartmentation of cholesterol in rat-liver microsomes, *Eur. J. Biochem.,* 34, 77, 1973.
134. **Bjorkhem, I. and Danielsson, H.,** 7α-hydroxylation of exogenous and endogenous cholesterol in rat-liver microsomes, *Eur. J. Biochem.,* 53, 53, 1975.
135. **Mitropoulos, K. A., Myant, N. B., Gibbons, G. F., Balasubramaniam, and Reeves, B. E. A.,** Cholesterol precursor pools for the synthesis of cholic and chenodeoxycholic acids in rats, *J. Biol. Chem.,* 249, 6052, 1974.
136. **Long, T. T., III, Jakoi, L., Stevens, R., and Quarfordt, S.,** The sources of rat biliary cholesterol and bile acid, *J. Lipid Res.,* 19, 872, 1978.
137. **Schwarz, C. C., Berman, M., Vlahcevic, R., Halloran, L. G., Gregory, D. H., and Swell, L.,** Multicompartmental analysis of cholesterol metabolism in man, characterization of the hepatic bile acid and biliary cholesterol precursor sites, *J. Clin. Invest.,* 61, 408, 1978.
138. **Gielen, J., Van Cantfort, J., Robaye, B., and Renson, J.,** Rat-liver cholesterol 7α-hydroxylase 3. New results about its circadian rhythm, *Eur. J. Biochem.,* 55, 41, 1975.
139. **Duane, W. C., Gilberstadt, M. L., and Wiegand, D. M.,** Diurnal rhythms of bile acid production in the rat, *Am. J. Physiol.,* 236, R175, 1979.
140. **Ericksson, S.,** Biliary excretion of bile acids and cholesterol in bile fistula rats. Bile acids and steroids, *Proc. Soc. Exp. Biol. Med.,* 94, 578, 1957.
141. **Shefer, S., Hauser, S., Lapar, V., and Mosbach, E. H.,** Regulatory effects of sterols and bile acids on hepatic 3-hydroxy-3-methylglutaryl CoA reductase and cholesterol 7α-hydroxylase in the rat, *J. Lipid Res.,* 14, 573, 1973.
142. **Stanley, M. M., Paul, D., Gacke, D., and Murphy, J.,** Effects of cholestyramine, metamucil, and cellulose on fecal bile salt excretion in man, *Gastroenterology,* 65, 889, 1973.
143. **Leveille, G. A. and Sauberlich, H. E.,** Mechanism of the cholesterol-depressing effect of pectin in the cholesterol-fed rat, *J. Nutr.,* 88, 209, 1966.
144. **Eastwood, M. A. and Hamilton, D.,** Studies on the adsorption of bile salts to nonabsorbed components of the diet, *Biochim. Biophys. Acta,* 152, 164, 1968.
145. **Serafin, J. A. and Nesheim, M. C.,** Influence of dietary heat-labile factors in soybean meal upon bile acid pools and turnover in the chick, *J. Nutr.,* 100, 786, 1970.
146. **Nath, M. C. and Brahmankar, D. M.,** Effect of vitamin B_{12}, on unsaturated fat and hydrolyzed glucosecycloacetate on bile acid excretion in experimental hyperlipemia, *Proc. Soc. Expl. Biol. Med.,* 108, 337, 1961.
147. **McGovern, R. F. and Quackenbush, F. W.,** Influence of dietary fat on bile acid secretion of rats after portal injection of (^{3}H)-cholesterol and (4-^{14}C) cholesterol esters, *Lipids,* 8, 473, 1973.

148. **Wilson, J. D. and Siperstein, M. D.,** Effect of saturated and unsaturated fats on fecal excretion of end products of cholesterol-4-^{14}C metabolism in the rat, *Am. J. Physiol.*, 196, 596, 1959.
149. **Tidwell, H. C., McPherson, J. C., and Burr, W. W., Jr.,** Effect of the saturation of fats upon the disposition of ingested cholesterol, *Am. J. Clin. Nutr.*, 11, 108, 1962.
150. **Miettinen, T. A.,** Clinical implications of bile acid metabolism in man, in *The Bile Acids,* Chemistry, Physiology, and Metabolism, Vol. 2, Nair, P. P. and Kritchevsky, D., Eds., Plenum Press, New York, 1973, 191.
151. **Nestel, P. J., Haverstein, N., Whyte, H. M., Scott, T. J., and Cook, L. J.,** Lowering of plasma cholesterol and enhanced sterol excretion with the consumption of polyunsaturated ruminant fats, *N. Engl. J. Med.*, 288, 379, 1973.
152. **Portman, O. W.,** Nutritonal influences on the metabolism of bile acids, *Am. J. Clin. Nutr.*, 8, 462, 1960.
153. **Miettinen, T. A.,** Effect of nicotinic acid on the fecal excretion of neutral sterols and bile acids, in *Metabolic Effects of Nicotinic Acid and Its Derivatives,* Gey, K. F. and Carlson, L. A., Eds., Hans Huber, Bern, 1971, 667.
154. **Ginter, E.,** Cholesterol: Vitamin C controls its transformation to bile acids, *Science,* 179, 702, 1973.
155. **Beher, W. T.,** Bile Acids. Chemistry and physiology of bile acids and their influence on atherosclerosis, in *Monographs on Atherosclerosis,* Vol. 6, Kritchevsky, D., Pollak, O. J., and Simms, H. S., Eds., S. Karger, Basel, 1976, 138.
156. **Bekersky, I. and Mosbach, E. H.,** Effect of hormones on bile acid metabolism, in *The Bile Acids,* Chemistry, physiology and metabolism, Vol. 2, Nair, P. P., and Kritchevsky, D., Eds., Plenum Press, New York, 1973, 249.
157. **Beher, W. T.,** Bile acids. Chemistry and physiology of bile acids and their influence on atherosclerosis, in *Monographs on Atherosclerosis,* Vol. 6, Kritchevsky, D., Pollak, O. J., and Simms, H. S., Eds., S. Karger, Basel, 1976, 184.
158. **Miettinen, T. A.,** Effect of drugs and bile acid and cholesterol excretion, in *Lipid Metabolism and Atherosclerosis,* Int. Congr. Ser. No. 283, Excerpta Medica, Amsterdam, 1973, 77.
159. **Encrantz, J. C. and Sjovall, J.,** On the bile acids in the duodenal contents of infants and children: Bile acids and steroids, 72, *Clin. Chim. Acta,* 4, 793, 1959.
160. **Poley, J. R., Dower, J. C., Owen, C. A., Jr., and Stickler, G. B.,** Bile acids in infants and children, *J. Lab. Clin. Med.*, 63, 838, 1964.
161. **Kroker, R., Anwer, M. S., and Hegner, D.,** The age dependence of bile acid metabolism in rats, *Exp. Gerontol.*, 7, 539, 1977.
162. **Hurza, Z. and Zbuzkova, V.,** Decrease of excretion of cholesterol during aging, *Exp. Gerontol.*, 8, 29, 1973.
163. **Uchida, K., Yasuhara, N., Kadowaki, M., Haruto, T., Takano, K., and Takeuchi, N.,** Age-related changes in cholesterol and bile acid metabolism in rats, *J. Lipid Res.*, 19, 544, 1978.
164. **Bartov, I., Henderson, G. R., and Reiser, R.,** Sex differences in steroid retention and excretion in rats fed cholesterol, *Nutr. Metabol.*, 17, 312, 1974.
165. **Engelberg, H.,** Short term studies of effect of heparin upon cholesterol excretion in man, *Proc. Soc. Exp. Biol. Med.*, 102, 364, 1959.
166. **Spritz, N., Ahrens, E. H., Jr., and Grundy, S.,** Sterol balance in man as plasma cholesterol concentrations are altered by exchanges of dietary fats, *J. Clin. Invest.*, 44, 1482, 1965.
167. **Miettinin, T. A., Pelkonen, R., Nikkila, E. A., and Heinonen, O.,** Low excretion of fecal bile acids in a family with hypercholesterolemia, *Acta Med. Scand.*, 182, 645, 1967.
168. **Eriksson, S.,** Bile acid pool in the rat, *Acta Physiol. Scand.*, 48, 439, 1960.
169. **Hellstrom, K., and Sjovall, J.,** Turnover of deoxycholic acid in the rabbit, *J. Lipid Res.*, 3, 397, 1962.
170. **Mosbach, E. H., Halpern, E., and Brunder, J.,** Sterol metabolism in the rabbit, *Fed. Proc.*, 15, 525, 1956.

Chapter 5

CHOLESTEROL BALANCE AND WHOLE BODY KINETICS

Jacqueline Dupont

TABLE OF CONTENTS

I. INTRODUCTION

The need for cholesterol in various tissue cells has been elaborated in earlier chapters. The concept of exchange of molecules in cells and ultimate excretion of the cyclopentanophenanthrene ring is well established. In the whole organism, particularly the human, it has been considered important to learn the origin and fate of cholesterol molecules in their life cycle in the body. All of the regulatory mechanisms described for synthesis, absorption, transport, catabolism, and excretion must be in synchrony to maintain appropriate concentrations of cholesterol in each tissue. With the knowledge of all these separate processes, it is still desirable to evaluate the status of the processes in the whole organism without destructive techniques.

The earliest type of experiment for this purpose was a simple chemical balance study. Later, use of radioisotopes was added and presently variations of chemical and radiochemical balance and kinetic studies are used either together or separately. The ultimate objectives of such studies are: (a) to ascertain whether there is physiologically normal cholesterol metabolism throughout the body; (b) if there is apparent abnormality, such as excessive serum cholesterol concentration, then the objective is to learn which of the regulatory processes is defective; and finally, (c) it is desired to be able to evaluate the effectiveness of intervention in metabolism in an effort to restore normalcy.

II. BALANCE STUDIES

A. Chemical Balance Studies

The simplest definition of a balance study is the difference between ingestion (I) and excretion (E).

$$I - E = \text{balance} \tag{1}$$

In cholesterol metabolism, this measurement usually accounts for fecal excretion of neutral and acidic steroids. If ingestion is zero, the figure indicates total synthesis, but if it is greater than zero, the questions of absorption and enterohepatic circulation (EHC) are raised.

The results of sterol balance studies (not total steroids) conducted prior to 1957 have been reviewed by Gould and Cook.[1] The subjects were varied in age, sex, health status, and race, and the amounts of cholesterol and fat consumed varied among the several experiments. The percent of cholesterol absorbed ranged between 13 and 75, based upon simple excretion data.

The difficulty of quantitation of fecal steroids made total steroid balance studies of questionable validity prior to the 1960s. Neutral sterol and steroid balance studies conducted between 1957 and 1964 have been reviewed by Ahrens et al.,[2,3] at the Rockefeller University. These authors summarize published data to indicate daily excretion of neutral sterol to be 193 to 1800 mg and bile acids to be 87 to 4000 mg in man. The variability is attributed to defects in methodology. By their methods, sterol excretion was 498 to 538 mg/day and bile acids 101 to 271 mg/day for four subjects fed cholesterol-free formula diets.

Urinary excretion of cholesterol is not negligible[4,5] and additionally, there is loss from desquamation of epithelial cells.[6] The urinary losses are seldom quantitated and are considered to be unimportant. This is a matter which deserves further study. The loss from skin was shown to be about 83 mg/day in normal subjects fed low or high cholesterol diets.[6]

The mechanisms of cholesterol absorption have been described in Chapter 3. Quan-

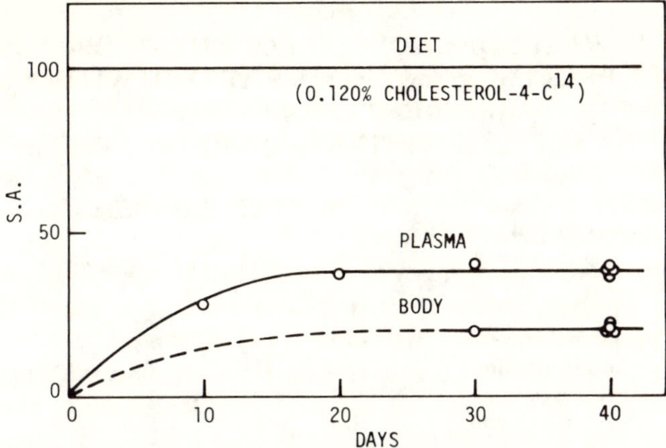

FIGURE 1. Example of isotopic equilibrium of cholesterol, following the ingestion of cholesterol-4-^{14}C. (From Chevallier, F., *Advances in Lipid Research,* Vol. 5, Paoletti, R. and Kritchevsky, D., Eds., 1967, 209. With permission.)

titation of absorption poses problems. It cannot be unequivocally determined by chemical balance techniques, so various combinations including radiochemical techniques have been introduced.

B. Radiochemical Balance Studies

1. Isotopic Steady State

Chevallier[4] began to use the isotopic steady state method in rats in 1956 and has reviewed studies conducted prior to 1967. His procedure involves feeding [^{14}C] cholesterol daily until the specific activities of plasma and tissue cholesterol reach plateau (Figure 1). This figure shows that 38% of the plasma cholesterol was labeled at the equilibrium state, therefore, it was of dietary origin. Combined with chemical balance data, the radiochemical data enabled Chevallier to obtain the results shown in Table 1. The fecal plus urinary excretion of neutral sterol equaled 3.0 mg/day while absorption equaled 1.5 mg/day when the rats were fed a diet containing 0.015% cholesterol. The total synthesis was 14.5 mg/day, but most of it was transformed (to bile acids). Increasing dietary cholesterol resulted in large increases in absorption, transformation and fecal and urinary excretion, and a small increase in synthesis.

Wilson[7] has used an isotopic steady state achieved by subcutaneous implantation of capsules containing [^{14}C] cholesterol and feeding [^{3}H] cholesterol. Results similar to those shown in Figure 1 were obtained. The fecal excretion of cholesterol by rats fed cholesterol-free diets was 2.5 mg/day and bile acids 3.5 mg/day. Feeding 0.5% cholesterol resulted in excretion of 2.2 mg/day of neutral sterol and 9.8 mg of bile acids. Wilson used a calculation of

$$\frac{[^{14}\text{C}] \text{ in fecal fraction (cpm)}}{\text{SA of blood cholesterol (cpm/mg)}} \qquad (2)$$

to determine mass of excretion (isotope balance method). Chevallier found that the SA of fecal cholesterol was not the same as that of blood cholesterol and, in fact, only one third was derived from subcutaneously administered or fed [^{14}C]-cholesterol.

Table 1
RATES OF CHOLESTEROL TURNOVER PROCESSES (mg/day) IN RATS FED WITH DIFFERENT CHOLESTEROL CONCENTRATION DIETS

Cholesterol turnover processes	Diet: cholesterol concentration 0.015	0.1	0.5	2.0
Absorption	1.5	12.8	49.6	100
Internal secretion	14.5	14.1	14.9	20.5
Transformation	13.2	21.1	55.2	99.5
Fecal excretion	2.5	2.7	5.0	12
Urinary excretion	0.5	1	1.1	9.5

From Chevallier, F., Advances in Lipid Research, Volume 5, Paoletti, R. and Kritchevsky, D., Eds., 1967, 209. With permission.

When dietary cholesterol was labeled with ^3H, Wilson found that bile acid excretion was 19.9 mg/day when 0.3% cholesterol was in the diet. The discrepancy between results using oral vs. subcutaneous cholesterol suggests that all the body cholesterol is not in equilibrium even over the time of these steady state experiments.

These experiments indicate that in the rat excess dietary cholesterol can be absorbed and then excreted as bile acids. The process requires several days to respond to increase in dietary cholesterol and can balance the excessive intake. These experiments require some contested assumptions for interpretation of results. Using only blood and fecal data, they do not reveal actual absorption vs. enterohepatic circulation, nor the origins of excreted cholesterol.

The isotopic steady state method was used for a study of human beings.[8] Cholesterol absorption was concluded to be quite low regardless of the amount in the diet. The calculations and assumptions used in interpreting the isotopic steady state have been discussed by Reiner.[9] He questioned the validity of the interpretations.

2. *Combination Methods*

a. Rats

Direct determinations of excretion and absorption of a single dose of radiolabeled cholesterol have been made. In rats, 45.3 to 53.4% of a tracer dose was excreted.[10] The amount absorbed was proportional to the amount fed (Figure 2). The absorption was verified by a subsequent study in which thoracic duct lymph was obtained by cannulation of the bile duct (Figure 3).[11] The rat appears to absorb 33 to 50% of dietary cholesterol regardless of amount consumed, the difference depending on the method of evaluation.

b. Humans

Studies of cholesterol balance have been complicated by difficulty of accurate quantitation of fecal sterols and steroids. Accurate analyses for fecal neutral and acidic steroids using gas-liquid chromatography and recovery of internal standards were validated in 1965.[2,3] The methods make chemical quantitation reliable. Quantitation of balances continues to present theoretical problems.

The first problem is transit time through the gastrointestinal tract. Various markers have been used to enable correlation of time of the period of ingestion of a particular diet with the excretion related to that time period. Chromic oxide has been validated

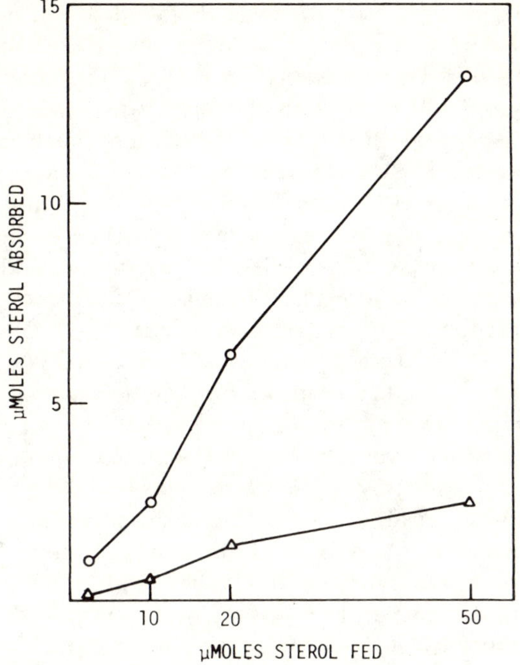

FIGURE 2. Total amounts of sterol present in the intestinal wall after feeding cholesterol. ○, cholesterol, △ sitosterol. (From Borgstrom, B., *J. Lipid. Res.*, 9, 474, 1968. With permission.)

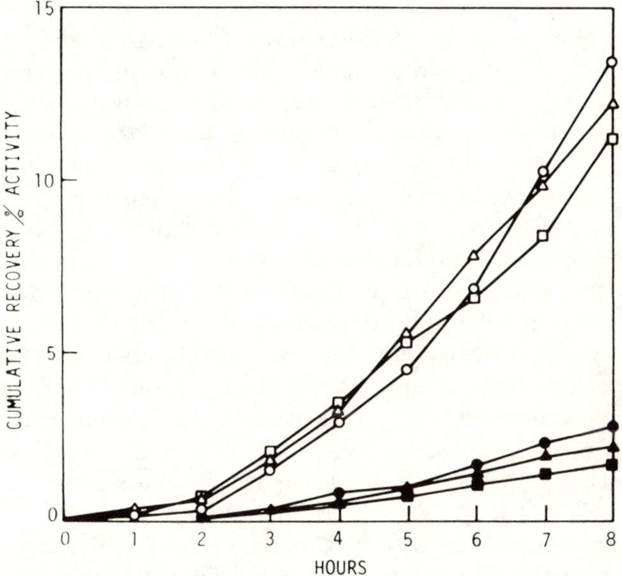

FIGURE 3. Cumulative percentage recoveries in thoracic duct lymph of labeled cholesterol (open symbols) and sitosterol (solid symbols) for the first 8 hr after feeding 0.03 µmol of cholesterol with 1.5 (○), 50 (△), and 100 (□) µmol of sitosterol in 800 µmol of triolein. (From Sylven, C. and Borgstrom, B., *J. Lipid Res.*, 10, 179, 1969. With permission.)

as suitable for that purpose.[12] The authors recommended that only subjects who excreted greater than 90% of the chromic oxide dose/day be included in balance studies. Twenty percent of their subjects sequestered the Cr_2O_3 in the colon.

Losses of neutral sterols during intestinal transit, which were considered to be unaccountable have been reported.[13,14] Labeled β-sitosterol has been considered to be a suitable nonabsorbable marker for sterols. The conviction that β-sitosterol is not absorbed is based upon reports of Gould[15] for man and Sylven and Borgstrom[11] for the rat. In fact, Gould[15] proved that β-sitosterol was absorbed by humans, incorporated into tissues, esterified and excreted via bile. The efficiency of absorption was about 10% of that of cholesterol in his subjects. Sylven and Borgstrom[11] showed 1.5 to 2.7% of fed sitosterol was transported to the lymph in the rat.

Other reports have indicated absorption of 22%,[16] 2 to 23%,[17] and 53%[18] of fed plant sterols by rats. These results were based on excretion of the unabsorbed material. Davignon et al.[12] reported failure of excretion of 8 to 43% of fed β-sitosterol by human subjects. The excretion pattern was not correlated with intestinal transit time.

The low concentration of β-sitosterol in plasma has been one reason absorption has been considered low. Salen et al.[19] concluded that about 10% of β-sitosterol was absorbed based upon measurements only of plasma concentration. It may be concluded that β-sitosterol disappears from the gut, enters the lymph, is incorporated into tissues, and excreted in bile in varying proportions of what is ingested. The appearance of plant sterols in skin is further confirmation of their absorption.[6]

The failure of loss of carbons from the ring structure of cholesterol was verified in 1952 by Chaikoff et al.[20] and has been reconfirmed by Chevallier.[4] In fact, intestinal bacterial degradation and carbon loss does not occur.[21,22] The germ-free baboon has been shown to excrete only about half the administered β-sitosterol determined either by recovery of mass or radioisotope.[23] In that experiment, the fecal recovery of cholesterol was about the same as that of sitosterol and neither was greatly affected by mono or polycontamination of the baboon's gastrointestinal tracts.

Use of β-sitosterol as a nonabsorbable marker is fallacious. The difference between ingested and excreted radiolabeled cholesterol is net absorption. What happens to the cholesterol which is not excreted must be accounted for. The use of radiolabeled cholesterol provides information on net absorption which adds to the information which may be derived from chemical balance methods. Still unaccounted for is the actual absorption and enterohepatic circulation of cholesterol when these methods are used.

In a study using swine, Marsh et al.[24] made an effort to resolve the problem of unaccountable loss of carbon from cholesterol in the intestinal tract. They found that by counting unextracted dried feces, plus all the radioactivity of sterols in tissues, they could account for all of the administered dose. In feces, the total radioactivity was not recovered in extracted neutral and acid sterols. The nonrecognizable steroid was presumed to come from neutral sterol breakdown, so the amount of neutral sterol accounted for as breakdown products was calculated by assuming that it had the same specific activity as the parent neutral sterol. Using these data, the authors concluded that it was not necessary to make corrections based upon a sterol marker such as β-sitosterol.

As in rats, human beings appear to absorb cholesterol in the range of 20 to 50% of that ingested regardless of the concentration in the diet (Figure 4).[25] Other studies have shown values of about 34 to 63% absorption (using β-sitosterol adjustments);[26] 0 to 53% absorption,[27] and 37 ± 5%,[28] and 42.3 ± 6.0% for cholesterol-free diet and 45.4 ± 8.3% following meals containing cholesterol.[29] Even though there have been reported wide ranges of individual variation and little significant treatment effects upon cholesterol absorption, the need to assess absorption as a part of the regulation of whole body metabolism of cholesterol continues.

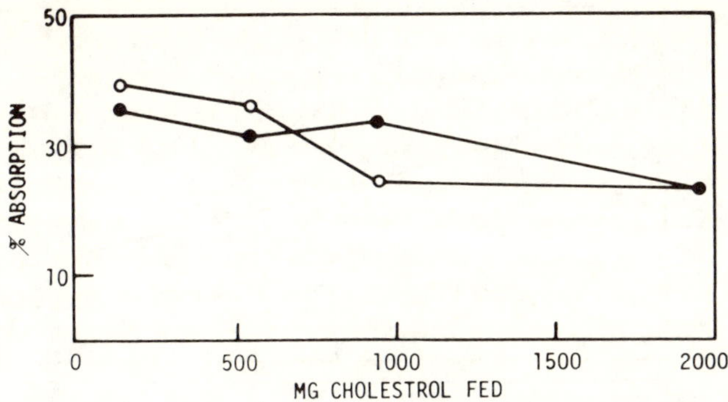

FIGURE 4. Apparent absorption of different doses of labeled cholesterol fed to humans in a single test meal. The figures have been calculated from fecal recoveries of activity over the 5 days succeeding the feeding. •; only cholesterol was fed and the recoveries were corrected by the use of an external standard in the form of B-sitosterol-22,23-^{3}H added to the feces. O; cholesterol-4-^{14}C was fed with 150 mg of B-sitosterol-22,23-^{3}H and the absorption figures were calculated by correction to a theoretical 100% sitosterol excretion. (From Borgstrom, B., *J. Lipid Res.*, 10, 331, 1969. With permission.)

A recent innovation in determination of cholesterol absorption in man has been the use of intestinal perfusion and sampling from lumen tubes situated at specific sites in the upper intestine.[30] This method may be used with radiotracer cholesterol and resulted in the observation that tracer and mass of cholesterol were not absorbed at the same rate. Using β-sitosterol adjustments, the authors reported percentage absorptions of 34 to 56.

Later studies using this method gave average absorptions of 63 ± 15 for normolipemic nonobese subjects, 59 ± 6 for obese, and 57 ± 11 for hyperlipemic subjects.[31] All subjects were adult Caucasians.

3. Plasma Isotope Ratio Method

A simpler method for determination of cholesterol absorption was proposed by Zilversmit for rats.[32] It involves simultaneous administration of [^{3}H] cholesterol orally and [^{14}C] cholesterol intravenously (or vice versa) and subsequent analysis of the ratio of ^{14}C and ^{3}H in serum cholesterol.

$$\frac{\text{Percentage of the oral dose in an aliquot of plasma}}{\text{Percentage of the intravenous dose in the same aliquot of plasma}} \times 100 \qquad (3)$$

In rats, the ratio was constant for several days after the first 24 hr, and indicated 48.5 ± 9.0% absorption vs. 44.1 ± 9.6% by the simple fecal loss method.

Subsequently, Zilversmit and Hughes[33] compared the plasma isotope ratio with fecal loss and with the ratio of the areas under the curves of 3-day disappearance data. The three methods agreed well and the isotope ratio gave values ranging from 36 to 58% absorption. This method has been used with apparent good results with miniature swine[34] to give a value of 41.5% absorption; squirrel, cebus, and rhesus monkeys to give values of 8.7 to 72% absorption;[35] vervet monkeys, 26.9%; baboons, 26.3% absorption.[36]

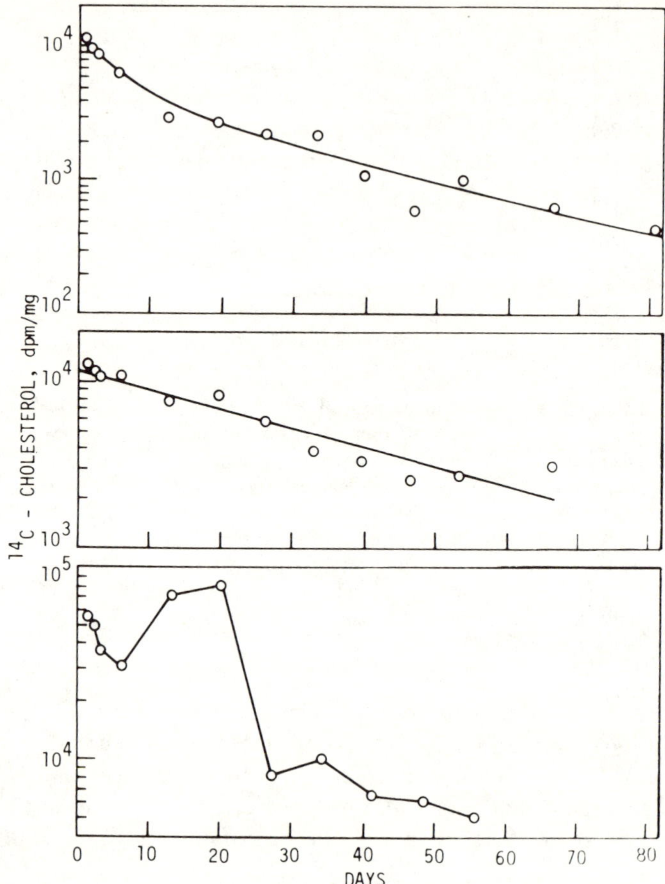

FIGURE 5. Disapperance of 4-^{14}C-cholesterol from the serum of foxhounds following i.v. injections. Examples of individual dogs exhibiting two-component, one-component and complex disappearance curves.

In human studies, the isotope ratio method has been carefully studied in comparison to fecal recovery methods.[37] The plasma isotope curves were parallel after 3 days and remained so for as long as 60 weeks. Three of 11 subjects were considered to be "technically unacceptable" because of low recovery of Cr_2O_3. Fortunately, the data were reported both with and without corrections. In the subjects having technically acceptable data, the fecal recovery and isotope ratio methods agreed extremely well. In the three aberrant subjects, the fecal recovery data gave much higher values when subjected to correction than were obtained with isotope ratio. In view of the need to identify abnormalities of cholesterol metabolism in individuals, it would seem that the aberrant subjects might be more interesting than the technically acceptable subjects, and the isotope ratio data considered to be of interest.

The ratio for only 3 days may not be sufficient for accurate analysis. Dogs do not seem to be amenable to this method unless the time is extended to 28 or more days and an area ratio used.[38] In that case, they were shown to absorb 56.5 ± 4.3% when fed a low cholesterol diet and 46.5 ± 4.0% when fed 1 to 5% cholesterol.

The reason the data for dogs were not suitable for simple plasma ratio calculations is illustrated in Figure 5.[38] Some portion of the injected dose was sequestered for several days in some animals. When it began to be released, the disappearance lines were not parallel. The isotope ratio data for the first few days were not in agreement with the area ratio determined after the slopes of the lines became constant. A similar condition may exist in the reports on primates.[35,36] These authors reported low fecal recovery of β-sitosterol and cholesterol. The apparent absorption indicated by fecal recovery of cholesterol was much higher than that indicated by the plasma isotope ratio. Some form of tissue sequestration of tracer doses apparently occurred. The conclusion as to percent absorption by monkeys and baboons is questionable until a longer disappearance curve is available. The fecal recovery indicating 80 to 90% absorption[35,36] appears to be the more valid measure.

The plasma isotope method is theoretically free of contestable assumptions. If the curves of disappearance are parallel, the ratio incontrovertibly indicates internal/external cholesterol. If the curves are not parallel, then one must simply wait until they have reached a steady decline and calculate the area ratio. The latter procedure was tested by Samuel et al.[37] and determined to be in close agreement with the plasma isotope ratio when the lines were parallel. Clearly, there is a need to account for the sequestration of tracer cholesterol and a genuinely physiological form of i.v. cholesterol developed.

C. Summary

The ultimate conclusion to be drawn from studies of cholesterol absorption is that it is not a major site of regulation of body cholesterol. Balance studies, whether chemical or radiochemical, indicate only net synthesis or loss of cholesterol from endogenous sources compared to diet. Balance studies must include quantitation of neutral and acidic steroid fractions to be informative. This can be done as illustrated by the Rockefeller University studies.[2,3] Those reports, which include neutral sterol data which have been altered in relation to less than 100% excretion of β-sitosterol rather than actual fecal recovery, cannot be interpreted as to steroid balance.

III. METABOLIC POOLS AND WHOLE BODY KINETICS

A. The Concept of Body Pools of Cholesterol

The first conception of body pools of cholesterol involved only endogenous and exogenous sources. The term pool means the total of a particular defined kind of cholesterol. With the use of radioisotope labeled cholesterol, the equilibration studies of Chevallier[4] indicated that not all the body cholesterol was exchangeable with the tracer cholesterol. Chevallier used the term "space of transfer" to describe the exchangeable pool. Data from experiments illustrated in Figure 1 indicated that the plasma cholesterol comes into equilibrium with dietary cholesterol at one level and plasma cholesterol is in equilibrium with body cholesterol at another level.

Labeling plasma cholesterol directly by intravenous injection has since become a common method for observing whole-body cholesterol kinetics. The disappearance of a single injected pulse of labeled cholesterol follows the pattern shown in Figure 6.[39] The pattern is very similar to that observed after daily feeding of labeled cholesterol is discontinued (Figure 7).[4] Such curves are interpreted to mean that each change of slope indicates a different kinetic pool or family of pools of cholesterol.

B. Mathematical Description of Kinetic Pools

The actual disappearance curve obtained is the average of several curves having different rates of exchange of cholesterol. The three component curve (Figure 6) is the average of three theoretical curves (Figure 8). These are described as three different pools, i.e., three kinds of cholesterol, but without ascribing any characteristics to them except their rate of exchange with plasma cholesterol. The three components of the

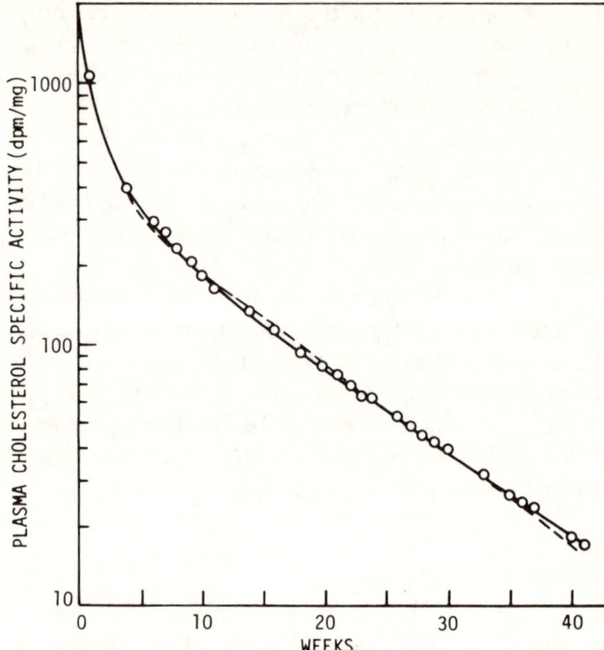

FIGURE 6. Computer analysis of the turnover of plasma cholesterol in a human subject. Observed data points are represented by circles. The solid curve represents the best fit to the data which can be obtained with a three-pool model, whereas the broken curve represents the best fit obtained with a two-pool model. (From Goodman, D. S., Noble, R. P., and Dell, R. B., *J. Lipid Res.*, 14, 178, 1973. With permission.)

curve are also referred to as describing compartments, which refers to location. Disappearance of labeled cholesterol provides the curves but does not define the characteristics of cholesterol within pools (i.e., free, esterified, protein bound) nor the location of the compartments (organ, subcellular).

The mathematical theory and derivation of equations for analyzing curves has been reviewed by Reiner[9] and explained by Shipley and Clark.[40] The commonly used principles of mathematical biology for cholesterol kinetics are precursor and product curves and compartmental analysis of disappearance curves. Figure 9[9] illustrates the theory that the specific activity-time curves of a precursor and product intersect at the maximum point of the product curve. Figure 10[9] shows the same situation if the labeled precursor has to penetrate the product compartment before the reaction could occur.

Curves may be obtained from complex systems which do not exhibit this theoretical configuration. Figure 11 illustrates such a possible curve. The actual cause of this is, a reaction chain has taken place $A'' \rightarrow A' \rightarrow A$ and only A'' and A have been measured. The theoretical complete picture is shown in Figure 8. The intermediate curve S' may indicate a chemical intermediate or an intermediate compartment, or perhaps both.

The situation where the product curve reaches its maximum before it intersects the precursor curve (Figure 12) indicates that a diluting reaction has occurred.[9] In the case of cholesterol transformations, it means that endogenously synthesized cholesterol is available to the reaction compartment.

When one has obtained a cholesterol disappearance curve by measuring the specific activity (SA) of plasma cholesterol following intravenous administration of the tracer, the first mathematical analysis is linearization of the components of the curve. This is often dubbed "curve peeling." Computerized systems for solving exponential func-

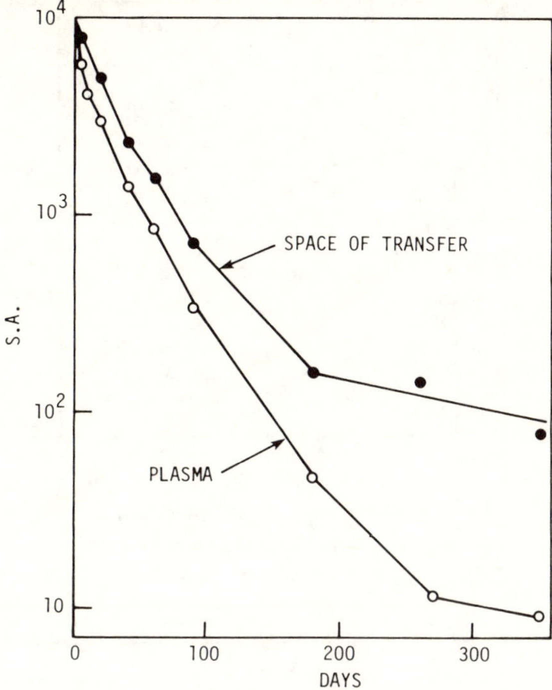

FIGURE 7. Decrease of plasma and body transfer cholesterol S.A. after 24 days of cholesterol-C^{14} feeding. (From Chevallier, F., *Advances in Lipid Research,* Volume 5, Paoletti, R. and Kritchevsky, D., Eds., 1967, 209. With permission.)

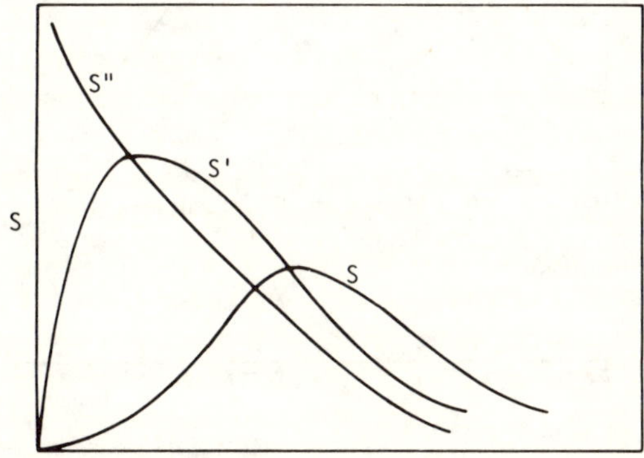

FIGURE 8. Hypothetical analysis of a three-component disappearance curve.

tions yield data for slopes and intercepts of each part of the linearized curve.

Early use of such data yielded only turnover time or half-life values.[41] That information has not been very informative, as the values tend to be similar for most species evaluated and for unpredictable and variable experimental and population variables within species (Table 2).

Use of compartmental models has been much more informative. One-pool, two-pool, and three-pool models have been devised. Figure 8 illustrates the curve analyses used for the calculations. Figure 13 shows the models depicted.

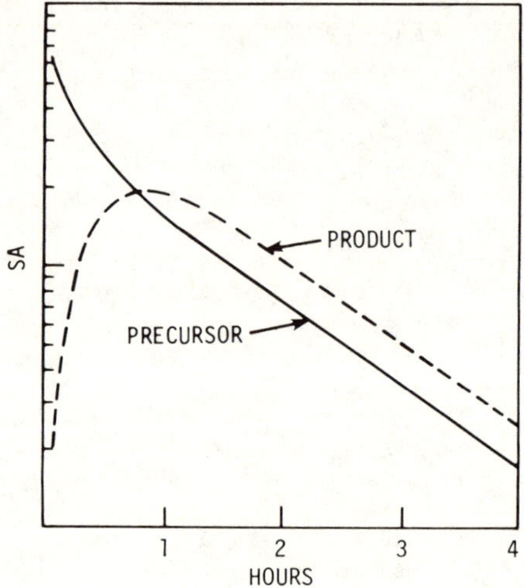

FIGURE 9. Hypothetical precursor-product curve.

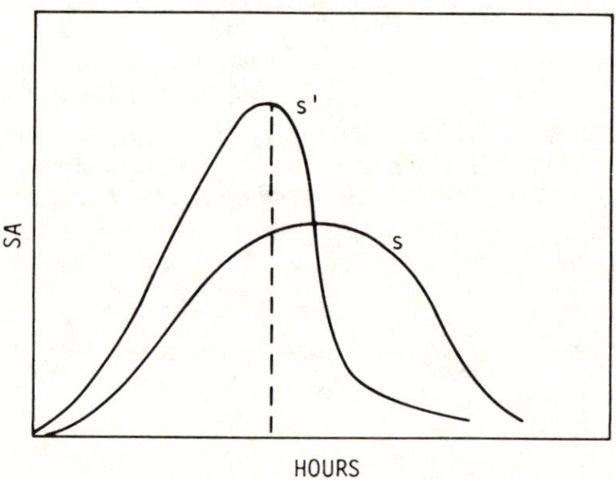

FIGURE 10. Hypothetical precursor product curve if precursor must penetrate the product compartment.

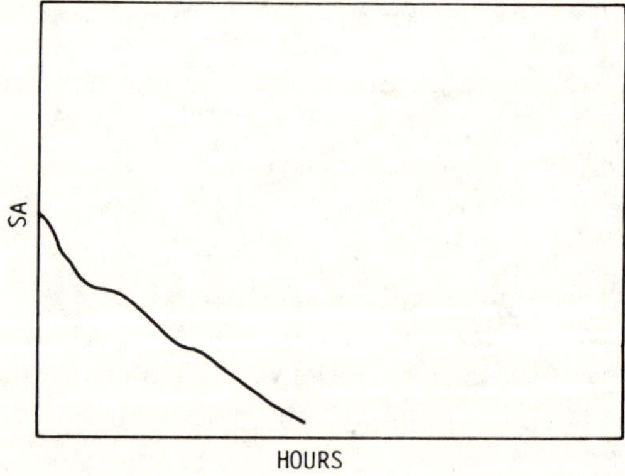

FIGURE 11. Possible curve obtained by measuring product of three-step reaction.

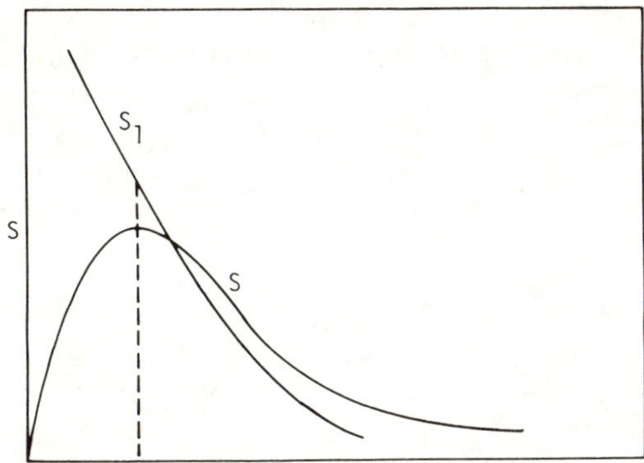

FIGURE 12. Hypothetical curve in which product is diluted after reaction.

Chobanian[48] used calculations from the flatest linear portion of a two-component curve to estimate whole body turnover (part A of Figure 13). Goodman and Noble[44] used both components of the curve to calculate parameters of a two-pool model (B, Figure 13). Goodman et al.[39] found that if they continued measuring plasma cholesterol SA for many months, some people would exhibit a three-compartment curve (C, Figure 13).

C. Physiological Interpretation of Pools

Assumptions which have been used in the two- and three-pool models are that pool 1 contains most of newly synthesized cholesterol (from gut and liver) and all dietary and enterohepatic cholesterol; pool 2 contains cholesterol more slowly exchangeable, probably muscle and adipose cholesterol; and pool 3 contains the very slowly exchanging cholesterol of brain and nervous tissue. Implicit in all the models is the knowledge that there is a pool which is not exchanging with serum cholesterol. These assumptions have been based upon studies of tissue cholesterol metabolism.

Figure 14 shows the disappearance of labeled cholesterol from tissues of rats following isotopic steady state labeling.[4] Data for brain are shown in Figure 15. Single isotope pulse administration to rats yielded data shown in Figure 16[49] and Figure 17.[45] Spleen and liver appear to be in constant equilibrium with serum. Heart and lung required several days to reach maximum SA (Figure 16) with maximum SA occurring after the product (tissue) line crossed the precursor (serum) line, indicating an intermediate compartment. Muscle (Figure 17) required 10 to 14 days to reach maximum SA which occurred at about the point of crossover with serum decline. The cholesterol SA in these tissues did not decrease in parallel with serum cholesterol as would be predicted by simple precursor-product kinetics. The SAs had an equilibrium configuration suggesting additional compartmentation within the tissue. Adipose tissue of the rat (Figure 17) acted as a sequestrant for the cholesterol dose, not reaching equilibrium with serum after 72 days.

Sequestration of labeled dose has been studied in rats.[50] In the first 24 hr particulate cholesterol is taken up by Kupfer cells of liver. In several studies, adipose tissue has displayed a higher specific activity than serum following administration of tracer cholesterol.[45,51,52] In most studies where tissues have been analyzed, the time points were infrequent. Figure 17[45] indicates that eventually the adipose tracer cholesterol disappears at a rate comparable to other tissues. The data in Figures 15 through 17 show that the tissues studied all contain two pools of cholesterol, comparable in turnover rates to the two pools shown by plasma analysis.

Additional results have been reported for rat leg muscle[53] with specific activity as a

Table 2
SPECIES COMPARISON OF T½ OF VARIOUS COMPONENTS DERIVED FROM SA OF CHOLESTEROL VERSUS TIME PLOTS

Species	Component 1 (days)	Component 2 (days)	Component 3 (days)	Ref.
Baboon	2.8-3.5	23—37		42
Baboon		47—56		43
Rhesus monkey		31—49		43
Squirrel monkey		17—20		43
Man	4-8.4	23—95		26
Man	3.33-6.35	25.2—85		44
Man	2.02-4.09	8.57—16.06	55.6-68.5	39
Rat	2.7	18.4		45
Miniature pig	2.66-4.21	14.3—25.2		34
Dog	1.6-3.3	11—35		46
Dog	4.59	22.93		38
Dog		9.2—63		47

plateau from about the fifth to ninth days. In both studies of muscle, the maximum of the muscle SA was to the right of the intersection with serum SA. The same has been reported for humans.[54] In precursor-product relationship, this indicates that there are intermediate pools between precursor and product.[9] The lifetime of the intermediate pool appears to be more than one week in these studies.

Studies in which arterial cholesterol has been measured, show it to have a slow turnover.[55,56] Dayton[55] has shown that the maximum SA of aorta cholesterol in cockerels occurs before intersection with the plasma SA curve. This deflection to the left indicates dilution of the label[9] which he interprets as local synthesis of as much as 20%, which is enough to negate the usual assumption about the two-pool model having no synthesis in pool 2.

In monkeys, Moutafis and Myant[56] have shown that muscle cholesterol SA peaks at the intersection with the plasma curve and subsequently decays with two components. Skin, on the other hand, had a peak prior to the intersection with plasma, indicating local synthesis, and a two-component disappearance rate as fast as plasma. Bhattacharya et al.[6] reported that surface skin lipid in normal human subjects reached peak SA after the intersection with plasma and had a slower disappearance thereafter. The abnormal situation of xanthoma cholesterol turnover has been studied by Bhattacharya et al.[57] It was found to be in rapid equilibrium with plasma, had a single component and $T_{1/2}$ between the slow and fast pools of plasma. Xanthoma cholesterol was concluded to have distinctly different metabolic characteristics than atheroma cholesterol.

D. Differentiation of Change and Abnormalities of Pools

Many studies have been directed to determining whether various experimental or therapeutic treatments would affect the parameters measured by turnover studies. Smith et al.,[58] using the three-pool model shown in Figure 13, found that pool sizes were related to body size and to serum lipids under different conditions of hyperlipemia (Table 3). Miller et al.[59] reported that pool sizes were related to total cholesterol in different lipoprotein classes. The size of pool 1 was positively correlated with body weight, while pool 2 was more closely related with excess body weight. When these relationships to body weight were taken into consideration, plasma total, very low density lipoprotein (VLDL), and low density lipoprotein (LDL), cholesterol concentrations were not correlated with body pool sizes, but there was a strong negative correlation between pool sizes and high density lipoprotein (HDL) concentration. Choles-

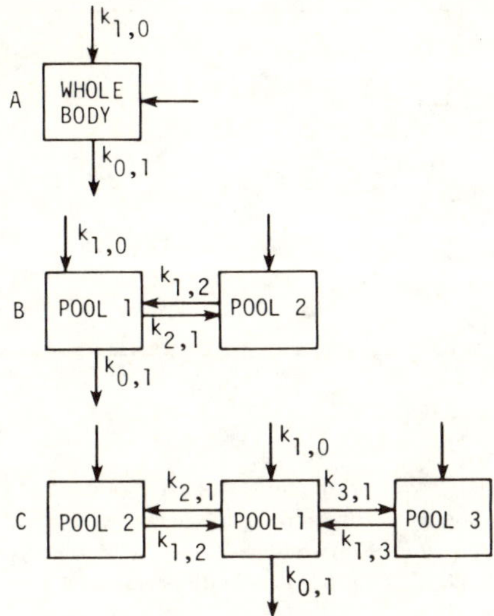

FIGURE 13. Hypothetical models of disappearance curves. A. single pool; B. 2 pool; C. 3 pool.

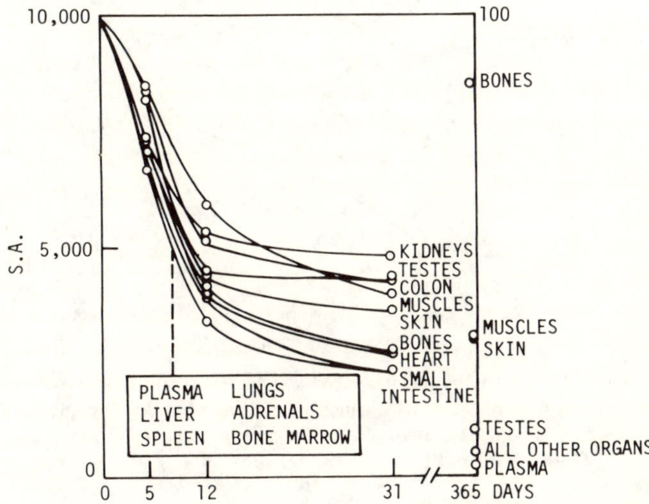

FIGURE 14. Decrease of plasma and organ transfer cholesterol SA after 24 days of cholesterol-C^{14} feeding. (From Chevallier, F., *Advances in Lipid Research,* Volume 5, Paoletti, R. and Kritchevsky, D., Eds., 1967, 209. With permission.)

terol turnover in patients with type II hypercholesterolemia and normal subjects was compared by Bhattacharya et al.[60] They found that pool size was affected by the lipid abnormality as shown in Table 4.

In the above-mentioned studies, the usual assumptions were made when the equations describing the two-pool model were formulated. All of the studies, however, were comparing normal subjects with genetically abnormal subjects. The degree of abnormality varied, but in type II hyperlipoproteinemia, it is not safe to assume that synthesis is negligible in pool 2 (see Chapter 3). The data could have been used to test for the possibility of synthesis.

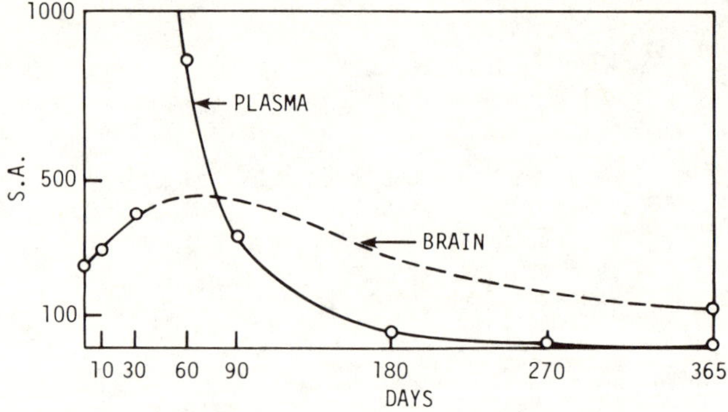

FIGURE 15. SA of brain cholsterol after 24 days of C^{14} cholesterol feeding as a function of time. (From Chevallier, F., *Advances in Lipid Research,* Volume 5, Paoletti, R. and Kritchevsky, D., Eds., 1967, 209. With permission.)

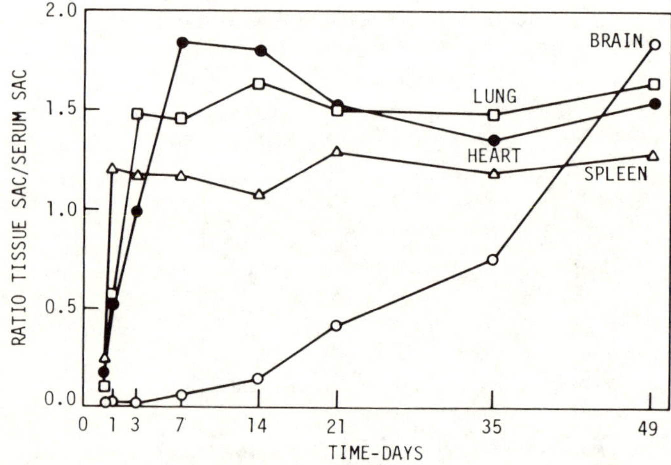

FIGURE 16. Ratio of specific activity (SAC) of tissue cholesterol to that of serum cholesterol as a function of time after feeding cholesterol-4-^{14}C. (From Chevallier, F., *Advances in Lipid Research,* Volume 5, Paoletti, R. and Kritchevsky, D., Eds., 1967, 209. With permission.)

Changes in the continuity of the disappearance curve have been observed when sudden changes in cholesterol metabolism were initiated. Clofibrate administration caused a decrease in rate of disappearance (Figure 18).[61,62] Change from 70% to 20% fat calories had a similar effect (Figure 19)[63] as did weight reduction (Figure 20).[64] The change in disappearance rate followed a sudden rise in serum cholesterol specific activity. The rise may result from a combination of serum cholesterol decrease and influx of cholesterol with higher specific activity from tissues.

E. Evolution of New Models

1. Background

The use of the three-pool model and all of its calculations and assumptions does not account for what is known about cholesterol metabolism. Balasubramaniam et al.[65] have shown that a pool of cholesterol in the liver which is accessible to 7-α-hy-

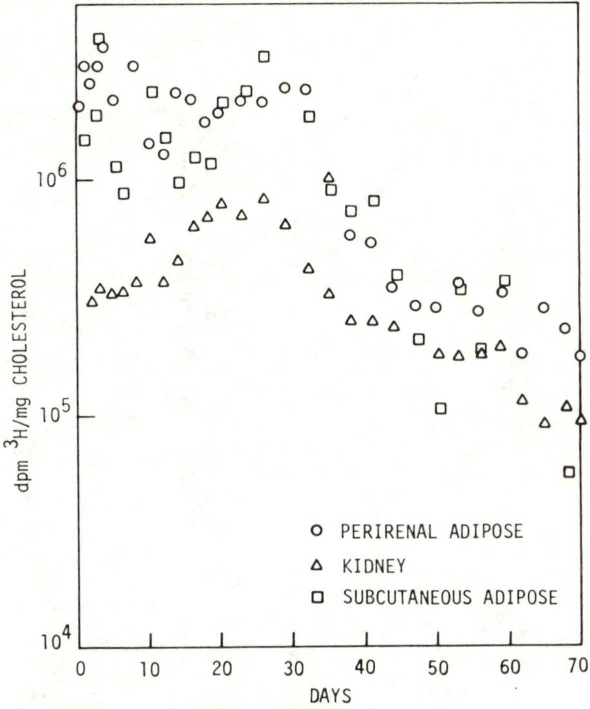

FIGURE 17. Appearance-disappearance of 1,2-^{3}H-cholesterol in serum, liver and skeletal muscle following intraperitoneal injection (each point represents the mean of 3-4 rats). (From Oh, S. Y., Dupont, J., and Clow, D. J., *Steroids*, 27, 637, 1976. With permission.)

droxylase does not account for the total cholesterol pool in the liver. Ogura et al.[66] have studied the cholesterol pool which acts as a precursor to bile acids. Using ring-labeled free cholesterol, esterified cholesterol, and cholesterol derived from labeled mevalonate (endogenous) in rats with bile fistulas, they reached the conclusion that liver free cholesterol is the precursor to bile acids. This would lead, by analogy with Balasubramaniam et al.,[65] to the conclusion that the 7-α-hydroxylase accessible pool is free cholesterol.

Mitropoulos et al.[67] have studied the EHC pool further. They conclude that the primary source for it is newly synthesized cholesterol. They used rats fed an essentially cholesterol free diet. The results add to support of a distinct pool of hepatic cholesterol accessible to cholic acid synthesis. In addition, they found that chenodeoxycholic acid may be formed from a different pool of cholesterol than that available for cholic acid synthesis. In agreement with the conclusion of Mitropoulos et al.,[67] Schwartz et al.[68] found that bile acids derived from infused mevalonate in man did not show a precursor-product relationship with plasma cholesterol or biliary cholesterol. On the contrary, Kim et al.[69] have concluded from data obtained in swine by entirely different experimental design that the bile acid precursor is a mixture of dietary and endogenously synthesized cholesterol.

2. Simulation Analysis and Modeling (SAAM)

A different method of examining kinetic data has been developed by Berman.[70] In this method, a model is designed using assumptions drawn from all the available knowledge of metabolism, and the model is tested by a simulation computer program[70]

Table 3
CHARACTERISTICS OF POPULATION GROUPS AND THEIR CHOLESTEROL KINETIC PARAMETERS.

Group (Number of Subjects)	Age (yr)	Height (cm)	Weight (kg)	Surface area (m^2)	Ideal body weight (%)	Excess weight (kg)	Serum Cholesterol (mg/dℓ)	Serum Triglyceride (mg/dℓ)
Normal (8)	39.4 ± 13.0	181 ± 6	76 ± 4	1.96 ± 0.09	102 ± 5	1.94 ± 3.29	204 ± 21	101 ± 20
Hypercholesterolemia (6)	54.5 ± 14.0	165 ± 11[b]	66 ± 19	1.73 ± 0.28	107 ± 11	4.69 ± 8.53	395 ± 94	120 ± 24
Mixed hyperlipidemia (8)	50.8 ± 8.5	174 ± 6	74 ± 12	1.87 ± 0.16	104 ± 10	3.35 ± 6.85	371 ± 89	306 ± 182
Hypertriglyceridemia (2)	57.5 ± 5.0	163 ± 25[a]	69 ± 7	1.74 ± 0.27	102 ± 3	1.42 ± 2.01	232 ± 12	255 ± 55
All subjects (24)	48.5 ± 12.8	173 ± 11	72 ± 12	1.85 ± 0.20	104 ± 8	3.05 ± 5.91	310 ± 110	187 ± 140

Note: Probability that value differs from normal by one-way analysis of variance and use of the Dunnett procedure (see Methods):

[a] $P < 0.05$
[b] $P < 0.01$

Subjects Studied by Groups: Unique Model Parameters (mean ± SD)

Group (Number of Subjects)	PR (g/day)	M_1 (g)	k_{12} (day^{-1})	k_{21} (day^{-1})	k_{13} (day^{-1})	k_{31} (day^{-1})	R_2 (g/day)	R_3 (g/day)
Normal (8)	1.14 ± 0.19	25.9 ± 2.8	0.071 ± 0.019	0.061 ± 0.015	0.018 ± 0.008	0.019 ± 0.014	1.57 ± 0.40	0.49 ± 0.35
Hypercholesterolemia (6)	0.98 ± 0.25	30.9 ± 8.6	0.079 ± 0.059	0.037 ± 0.013[a]	0.016 ± 0.005	0.021 ± 0.011	1.14 ± 0.59	0.68 ± 0.42
Mixed hyperlipidemia (8)	1.19 ± 0.28	28.4 ± 4.4	0.073 ± 0.037	0.044 ± 0.014[c]	0.017 ± 0.007	0.026 ± 0.014	1.23 ± 0.39	0.73 ± 0.34
Hypertriglyceridemia (2)	1.01 ± 0.28	20.1 ± 0.6	0.193 ± 0.022[b]	0.075 ± 0.018	0.026 ± 0.002	0.048 ± 0.005	1.51 ± 0.31	0.97 ± 0.07
All subjects (24)	1.11 ± 0.25	27.5 ± 5.8	0.084 ± 0.050	0.050 ± 0.007	0.018 ± 0.007	0.025 ± 0.015	1.35 ± 0.46	0.66 ± 0.36

Note: Probability that value differs from normal by one-way analysis of variance and use of the Dunnett procedure (see Methods). Terms are defined in Figure 13. Subjects studied by groups: physiological variables (mean ± SD)

[a] $P < 0.05$
[b] $P < 0.01$
[c] $0.05 < P < 0.06$

From Smith, F. R., Dell, R. B., Noble, R. P., and Goodman, D. S., *J. Clin. Invest.*, 57, 137, 1976. With permission.

Table 4
DESCRIBING RESULTS OF CHOLESTEROL KINETIC STUDIES

	g/kg body weight					
	Isotopic cholesterol given IV			Isotopic cholesterol given orally		
	Normal	Type II	P-value	Normal	Type II	P-value
M_{AP}[b]	0.089 ± 0.013	0.212 ± 0.081	<0.005	0.089 ± 0.013	0.212 ± 0.081	<0.005
M_{AX}[b]	0.287 ± 0.036	0.512 ± 0.184	<0.025	0.360 ± 0.048	0.758 ± 0.348	<0.025
M_A[c]	0.377 ± 0.034	0.723 ± 0.214	<0.005	0.457 ± 0.035	0.969 ± 0.378	<0.01
M_B[d]	0.904 ± 0.277	1.097 ± 0.597	NS	0.968 ± 0.160	1.614 ± 1.156	NS
$M_A + M_B$[c]	1.281 ± 0.300	1.820 ± 0.760	NS	1.425 ± 0.180	2.583 ± 1.483	NS

[a] Total plasma pool, plasma cholesterol in milligrams per milliliter × total plasma volume calculated as 40 mℓ/kg body weight.
[b] $M_A - M_{AP}$, cholesterol pool of tissues comprising pool A, M_A.
[c] Pool size A, M_A.
[d] Pool size B, M_B.
[e] Total exchangeable pool, $(M_A + M_B)$.

From Bhattacharya, A. K., Conner, W. E., Mausolf, F. A., and Flatt, A. E., *J. Lab. Clin. Med.*, 88, 503, 1976. With permission.

to determine whether the data fit. This process takes account of the complexity of metabolism even though one or more linear 2-component disappearance curves constitute the available data.

The SAAM process can be used to integrate several sets of data for the same system. For cholesterol metabolism, Schwartz et al.[71] have analyzed serum and bile cholesterol and bile acids simultaneously. They have proposed a model shown in Figure 21. The data were obtained with human subjects, and the following assumptions were made:

1. The patients were in a steady state of cholesterol metabolism.
2. The patients had a total bile fistula, therefore there was no enterohepatic circulation of steroids.
3. Cholesterol from peripheral tissues must enter the plasma before entering the hepatocyte.
4. Bile represents the only significant pathway of loss of cholesterol from the body.

The constraint of the bile fistula limits the contribution of this study to the assignment of precursor pools for bile steroids. The next level of complication in modeling whole body metabolism requires additional data and additional assumptions. A preliminary model using data obtained in experiments with miniature swine has been developed.[72] The data consisted of serum and bile cholesterol disappearance from i.v. [^{14}C] cholesterol and bile acid appearance and disappearance (Figure 22).

A model was constructed based upon that developed by Schwartz[71] (Figure 23). The serum curve was analyzed and subsequently used as a forcing function (pool 4) to which the other data were fit (Figure 24). Pool X depicts the rapid sequestration and subsequent release of tracer cholesterol in the first few hours after injection. Pool 2 represents bile acid precursor cholesterol as measured by intestinal bile acid specific activity. Both Schwartz et al.[71] and Clow et al.[72] find this pool to be best represented by unidirectional flow (Figure 25). Pool 3 depicts bile cholesterol derived from serum cholesterol tracer. In the intact animal, the possibility of both exchange between liver and serum directly, and of enterohepatic circulation is present. In the Clow et al. model, the fit was best if exchange was assumed to take place (Figure 26).

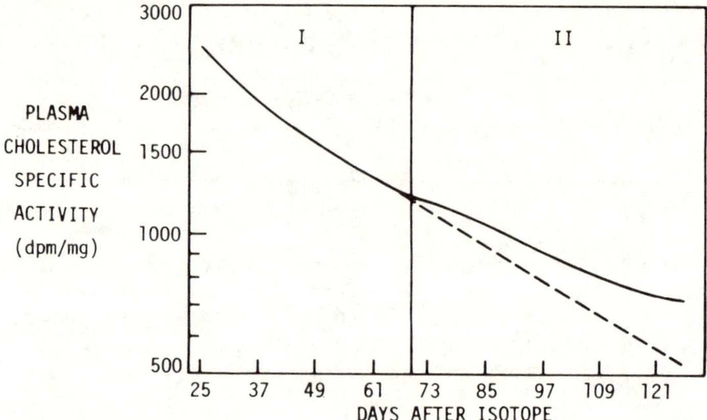

FIGURE 18. Cholesterol disappearance curve of human subject. Solid line indicates change in curve as a result of ingestion of clofibrate. (From Grundy, S. M., Ahrens, E. H., Jr., Salen, G., Schreibman, P. H., and Nestel, P. J., *J. Lipid Res.*, 13, 531, 1972. With permission.)

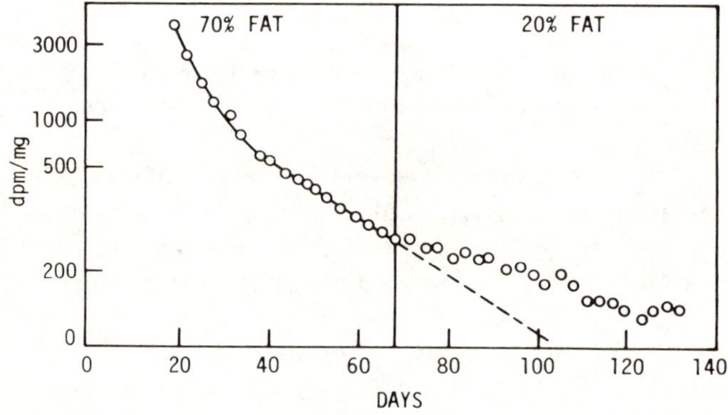

FIGURE 19. Cholesterol disappearance in a human subject. Vertical line indicates change in relation to quantity of fat consumed. (From Schreibman, P. H. and Ahrens, E. H., Jr., *J. Lipid Res.*, 17, 97, 1976. With permission.)

Schwartz et al.[71] had not assumed exchange of pool 3 with serum cholesterol. Some pool of cholesterol other than newly synthesized must be present because there is reappearance of labeled cholesterol in very low density lipoprotein (VLDL) continually up to 35 days after injection of tracer cholesterol.[73] Exchange among lipoproteins in serum should not be the only mode of incorporation of "old" cholesterol in VLDL.

Pool 6 is hypothesized in the model and can be simulated kinetically (Figure 27). It has a rapid rise and slow decay analogous to a slow and a fast pool as shown in tissues analyzed in other experiments (Figure 17).

The fits of pools 2 and 3 hypothetical curves to actual data are not perfect, although reasonably good. There is a need to conduct additional experiments to identify free and esterified cholesterol pools, kinetics of peripheral tissue pools, and further identification of cholesterol compartmentation in the liver where the exchange among pools has the greatest likelihood of occurring.

An additional pool in extrahepatic tissue may be postulated. The pool may represent esterified cholesterol in peripheral tissues. Results reported for metabolism of low den-

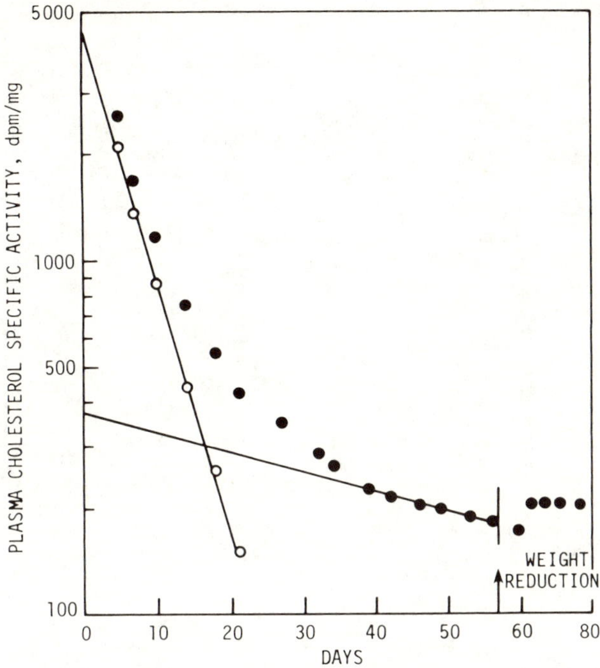

FIGURE 20. Semilogarithmic plot of plasma cholesterol specific activity vs. time in days in a typical obese patient. Body weight and calorie intake remained constant through 57 days of study at which time calorie intake was reduced by 80%. Note the sudden rise in the decay curve when weight reduction began. (From Nestel, P. J., Schreibman, P. H., and Ahrens, E. H., Jr., *J. Clin. Invest.*, 52, 2389, 1973. With permission.)

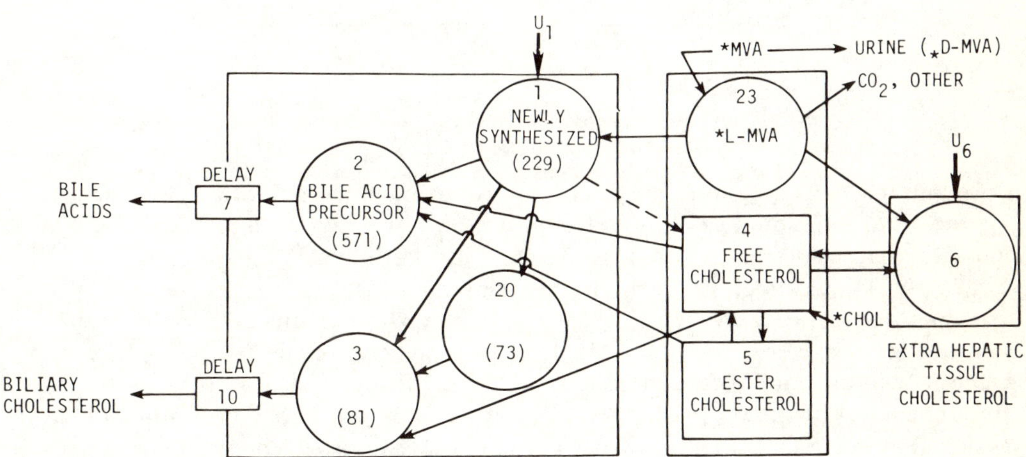

FIGURE 21. Model of cholesterol metabolism of Schwartz, et al.[71] Numbers in parentheses are representative values of calculated compartment size in micromoles from one patient.

sity lipoprotein (LDL) in cultured cells[74] suggest that esterification of cholesterol following entrance of LDL and hydrolysis in liposomes occurs. This pool of cholesterol may represent a slowly exchanging tissue pool. Tissues in rats have been reported to have both rapid and slowly exchanging pools of cholesterol.[45]

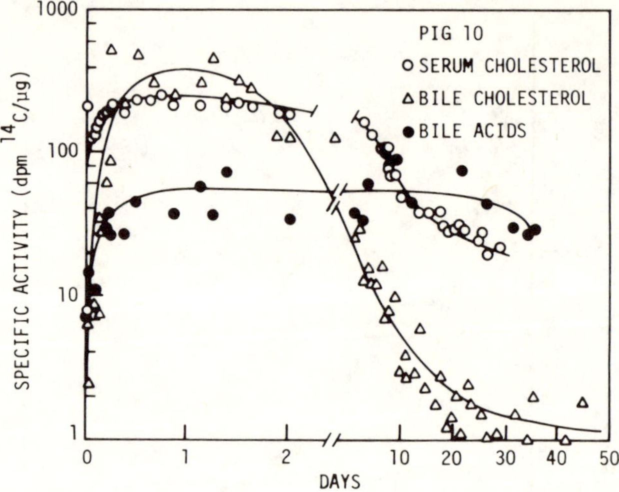

FIGURE 22. Kinetics of serum cholesterol disappearance and appearance as bile cholesterol and bile acids in miniature swine.[72]

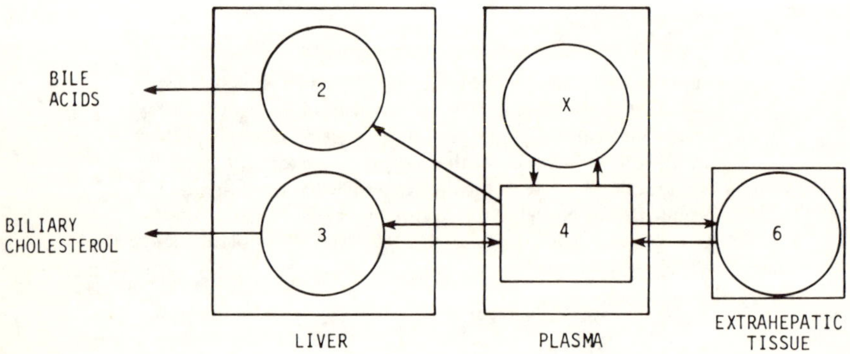

FIGURE 23. Proposed model of cholesterol metabolism.

Serum and bile cholesterol do not necessarily come into equilibrium. Bile acid formation from cholesterol exhibits a lag phase shown by a two-week plateau in SA. This indicates that the precursor pool is not in rapid equilibrium with the tracer.

The physiological compartmentation of slow and fast pools of cholesterol is proposed as shown in Figure 28. The fast pool is the cholesterol which cycles from the gut through the liver (path 1) and the liver to peripheral tissues (path 2) where it exchanges with the pool of free cholesterol of the tissue and returns to the liver (path 3). Enterohepatic circulation of cholesterol is part of this fast pool constituting a "short cycle" (paths 1 and 4). The slow pool is that cholesterol which enters the esterified cholesterol pool of peripheral tissues (path 5). This cholesterol must undergo hydrolysis before it can reenter the route of return to the liver for excretion or reentry into the fast pool. Newly synthesized cholesterol may enter either pool; the rates of synthesis and transport and esterification being too rapid to be resolved by kinetics of serum cholesterol disappearance.

Interpretation of disappearance kinetics for this hypothetical model is as follows. The fast pool is defined by the parameters of the fast component of the serum curve. Disagreement between the kinetics of the serum and bile fast curves indicates separa-

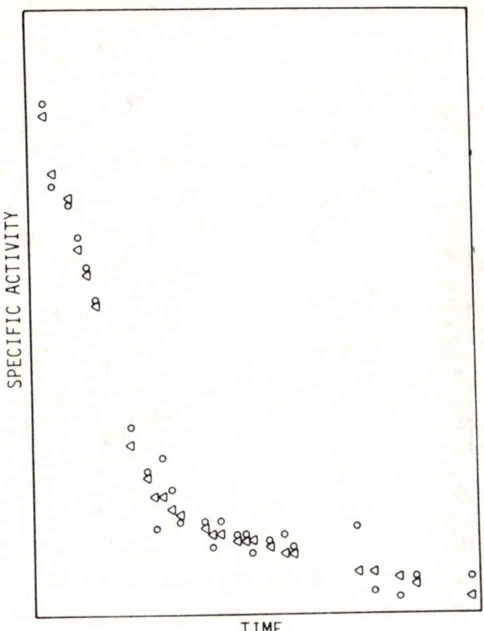

FIGURE 24. Serum cholesterol disappearance in a miniature pig. O are actual data points for cholesterol specific activity and Δ are fit by SAAM. Pool 4 of Figure 23.

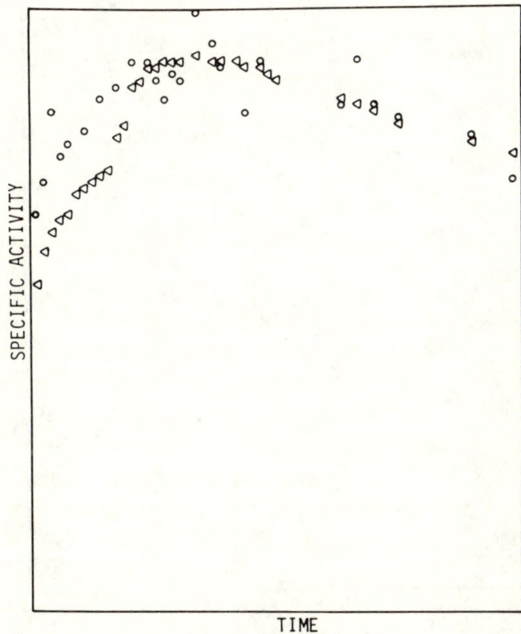

FIGURE 25. Bile acid appearance-disappearance in the intestine of a miniature pig O are actual data points for cholesterol specific activity and Δ are fit by SAAM. Pool 2 of Figure 23.

tion of the enterohepatic cycle (short cycle) from the complete cycle to peripheral tissues. The slow pool parameters describe the rate of equilibrium of free and esterified

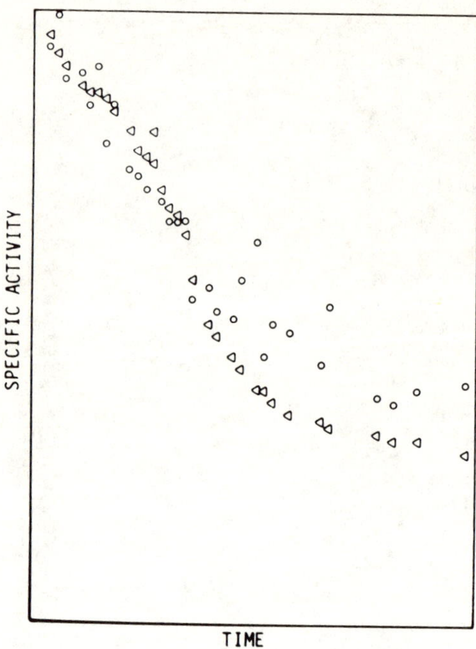

FIGURE 26. Bile cholesterol appearance-disappearance in the intestine of a miniature pig. O are actual data points for specific activity and △ are fit by SAAM. Pool 3 of Figure 23.

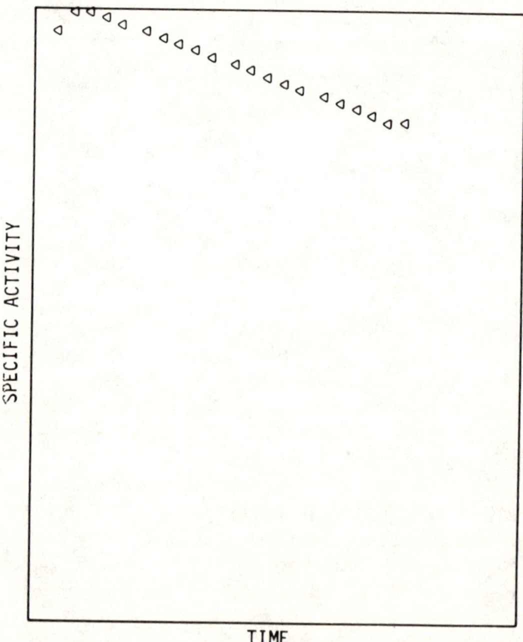

FIGURE 27. Hypothetical appearance-disappearance of cholesterol in peripheral tissues based upon data in Figures 24 through 26. Pool 6 of Figure 23.

cholesterol in peripheral tissues. This rate may account for the plateau of bile acid SA during the period of time when the fast and slow curves are not clearly resolved.

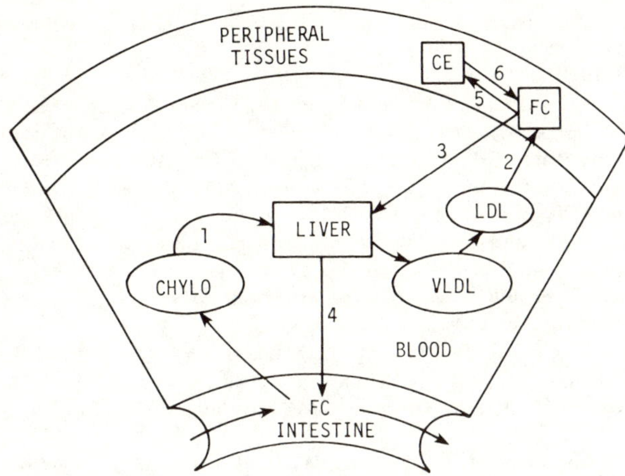

FIGURE 28. Proposed physiological compartmentation of cholesterol. FC is free cholesterol, CE is esterified cholesterol, VLDL is very low density lipoprotein cholesterol, LDL is low density lipoprotein cholesterol.

F. Summary

Cholesterol balance continues to be a useful concept in evaluation of whole body cholesterol metabolism. The problems of accounting for synthesis and recycling have not been resolved satisfactorily. This makes it impossible to accurately assess the mass of cholesterol absorbed in a period of time. Even the estimation of fractions of the available enteric cholesterol absorbed is subject to problems of assurance that a tracer is adequately reflecting the tracee cholesterol. Kinetic analysis of tracer cholesterol is a powerful tool which offers a method for testing assumptions, and with the use of stimulation analysis can allow extraction of more information from data.

REFERENCES

1. **Gould, R. G. and Cook, R. P.,** Metabolism of cholesterol and other sterols, in *Cholesterol,* Cook, R. P., Ed., Academic Press, New York, 1958, 237.
2. **Miettinen, T. A., Ahrens, E. H., Jr., and Grundy, S. M.,** Quantitative isolation and gas-liquid chromatogrphic analysis of total dietary and fecal neutral steroids, *J. Lipid Res.,* 6, 411, 1965.
3. **Grundy, S. M., Ahrens, E. H., Jr., and Miettinen, T. A.,** Quantitative isolation and gas-liquid chromatograhic analysis of total fecal bile acids, *J. Lipid Res,* 6, 397, 1965.
4. **Chevallier, F.,** Dynamics of cholesterol in rats, studied by the isotopic equilibrium method, in *Advances in Lipid Research,* Vol. 5, Paoletti, R. and Kritchevsky, D., Eds., 1967, 209.
5. **Nicholas, H. J.,** Bile acids and brain, *The Bile Acids,* Vol. 3: Pathophysiology, Nair, P. P. and Kritchevsky, D., Eds., Plenum Press, New York, 1976, 1.
6. **Bhattacharya, A. K., Connor, W. E., and Spector, A. A.,** Excretion of sterols from the skin of normal and hypercholesterolemic humans, *J. Clin. Invest.,* 51, 2060, 1972.
7. **Wilson, J. D.,** The quantification of cholesterol excretion and degradation in the isotopic steady state in the rat: The influence of dietary cholersterol, *J. Lipid Res.,* 5, 409, 1964.
8. **Wilson, J. D. and Lindsey, C. A., Jr.,** Studies on the influence of dietary cholesterol on cholesterol metabolism in the isotopic steady state in man, *J. Clin. Invest.,* 44, 1805, 1965.
9. **Reiner, J. M.,** Isotopic analysis of metabolic systems, Part I., *Exp. Mol. Path.,* 20, 78, 1974.
10. **Borgstrom, B.,** Quantitative aspects of the intestinal absorption and metabolism of cholesterol and β-sitosterol in the rat, *J. Lipid Res.,* 9, 474, 1968.
11. **Sylven, C. and Borgstrom, B.,** Absorption and lymphatic transport of cholesterol and sitosterol in the rat, *J. Lipid Res.,* 10, 179, 1969.

12. **Davignon, J., Simmonds, W. J., and Ahrens, E. H., Jr.,** Usefulness of chromic oxide as an internal standard for balance studies in formula-fed patients and for assessment of colonic function, *J. Clin. Invest.*, 47, 127, 1968.
13. **Grundy, S. M., Ahrens, E. H., Jr., and Salen, G.,** Dietary β-sitosteral as an internal standard to correct for cholesterol losses in sterol balance studies, *J. Lipid Res.*, 9, 374, 1968.
14. **Grundy, S. M. and Ahrens, E. H., Jr.,** Measurements of cholesterol turnover, synthesis, and absorption in man, carried out by isotope kinetic and sterol balance studies, *J. Lipid Res.*, 10, 91, 1969.
15. **Gould, R. G.,** Absorbability of beta-sitosterol, *N. Y. Acad. Sci. Trans.*, 18, 129, 1956.
16. **Ivy, A. C., Lin, T. M., and Karvinen, E.,** Absorption of dihydrocholesterol and soya sterols by the rat's intestine, *Am. J. Physiol.*, 193, 79, 1955.
17. **Swell, L., Boiter, T. A., Field, H., Jr., and Treadwell, C. R.,** The absorption of plant sterols and their effect on serum and liver sterol levels, *J. Nutr.*, 58, 385, 1956.
18. **Swell, L., Trout, E. C., Jr., Vahouny, G. V., Field, H., Jr., Von Schuching, S., Treadwell, C. R.,** Influence of ^{3}H-β-sitosterol on sterol excretion, *Proc. Soc. Exp. Biol. Med.*, 97, 337, 1958.
19. **Salen, G., Ahrens, E. H., Jr., and Grundy, S. M.,** Metabolism of β-sitosterol in man, *J. Clin. Invest.*, 49, 952, 1970.
20. **Chaikoff, I. C., Siperstein, M. D., Dauben, W. G., Bradow, H. L., Eastham, J. R., Tomkins, G. M., Meier, J. T., Chen, R. W., Hotta, S., and Srere, P. A.,** [^{14}C] cholesterol II. Oxidation of carbons 4 and 26 to carbon dioxide by the intact rat, *J. Biol. Chem.*, 194, 413, 1952.
21. **Wood, P. D. S. and Hatoff, D.,** Incubation of human fecal homogenates with 4 [^{14}C] cholesterol, *Lipids*, 5, 702, 1970.
22. **Levitt, M. D., Hanson, R. F., Bond, J. H., and Engel, R. R.,** Failure to demonstrate degradation of 4 [^{14}C] cholesterol to volatile hydrocarbons in rat and human fecal homogenates, *Lipids*, 10, 662, 1975.
23. **Mott, G. E., Roberts, C. J., Eichberg, J. W., McGill, H. C., Jr., and Kolter, S. S.,** Neutral steroid losses and cholesterol absorption in gnotobiotic baboons, *Exp. Mol. Path.*, 24, 333, 1976.
24. **Marsh, A., Kim, D. N., Lee, K. T., Reiner, J. M., and Thomas, W. A.,** Cholesterol turnover, synthesis, and retention in hypercholesterolemic growing swine, *J. Lipid Res.*, 13, 600, 1972.
25. **Borgstrom, B.,** Quantification of cholesterol absorption in man by fecal analysis after the feeding of a single isotope-labeled meal, *J. Lipid Res.*, 10, 331, 1969.
26. **Grundy, S. M. and Ahrens, E. H., Jr.,** Measurements of cholesterol turnover, synthesis, and absorption in man, carried out by isotope kinetic and sterol balance methods, *J. Lipid Res.*, 10, 91, 1969.
27. **Quintao, E., Grundy, S. M., and Ahrens, E. H., Jr.,** An evaluation of four methods for measuring cholesterol absorption by the intestine in man, *J. Lipid Res.*, 12, 221, 1971.
28. **Kudchodkar, B. J., Sodhi, H. S., Horlick, L.,** Absorption of dietary cholesterol in man, *Metabolism*, 22, 155, 1973.
29. **Connor, W. E. and Lin, D. S.,** The intestinal absorption of dietary cholesterol by hypercholesterolemic (Type II) and normoholesterolemic humans, *J. Clin. Invest.*, 53, 1062, 1974.
30. **Grundy, S. and Mok, H. Y. I.,** Determination of cholesterol absorption in man by intestinal perfusion, *J. Lipid Res.*, 18, 263, 1977.
31. **Mok, H. Y. I., von Bergmann, K., and Grundy, L. M.,** Effects of continuous and intermittent feeding on biliary lipid outputs in man: Application for measurements of intestinal absorption of cholesterol and bile acids, *J. Lipid Res.*, 20, 389, 1979.
32. **Zilversmit, D. B.,** A single blood sample dual isotope method for the measurement of cholesterol absorption in rats, *Proc. Soc. Exp. Biol. Med.*, 104, 862, 1972.
33. **Zilversmit, D. B., and Hughes, L. B.,** Validation of a dual-isotope plasma ratio method for measurement of cholesterol absorption in rats, *J. Lipid Res.*, 15, 465, 1974.
34. **Dupont, J., Oh, S. Y., O'Deen, L., McClellan, M. A., Lumb, W. V., and Butterfield, A. B.,** Cholesterol and bile acid turnover in miniature swine, *Lipids*, 9, 717, 1974.
35. **Corey, J. E. and Hayes, K. C.,** Validation of the dual-isotope plasma ratio technique as a measure of cholesterol absorption in old and new world monkeys, *Proc. Soc. Exp. Biol. Med.*, 148, 842, 1975.
36. **Kritchevsky, D., Winter, P. A. D., and Davidson, L. M.,** Cholesterol absorption in primates as determined by the Zilversmit isotope ratio method, *Proc. Soc. Exp. Biol. Med.*, 147, 464, 1974.
37. **Samuel, P., Crouse, J. R., and Ahrens, E H., Jr.,** Evaluation of an isotope ratio method for measurement of cholesterol absorption in man, *J. Lipid Res.*, 19, 82, 1978.
38. **Dupont, J., Nelson, A. W., and Clow, D. J.,** Cholesterol kinetics in control and hypercholesterolemic foxhounds, (Unpublished).
39. **Goodman, D. S., Noble, R. P., and Dell, R. B.,** Three-pool model of the long-term turnover of plasma cholesterol in man, *J. Lipid Res.*, 14, 178, 1973.
40. **Shipley, R. A. and Clark, R. E.,** *Tracer methods for in vivo kinetics*, Academic Press, New York, 1972.
41. **Zilversmit, D. B., Entenmann, C., and Fishler, M. D.,** The calculation of "turnover rate" from experiments involving the use of labeling agents, *J. Gen. Physiol.*, 26, 325, 1943.

42. **Wilson, J. D.**, The measurement of the exchangeable pools of cholesterol in the baboon, *J. Clin. Invest.*, 49, 655, 1970.
43. **Eggen, D. A.**, Cholesterol metabolism in rhesus monkey, squirrel monkey, and baboon, *J. Lipid Res.*, 15, 139, 1974.
44. **Goodman, D. S. and Noble, R. P.**, Turnover of plasma cholesterol in man, *J. Clin. Invest.*, 47, 231, 1968.
45. **Oh, S. Y., Dupont, J., and Clow, D. J.**, Kinetic analysis of cholesterol turnover in rat tissues, *Steroids*, 27, 637, 1976.
46. **Pertsemlidis, D., Kirtchman, E. H., and Ahrens, E. H., Jr.**, Regulation of cholesterol metabolism in the dog. II. Effects of complete bile diversion and of cholesterol feeding on absorption, synthesis, accumulation and excretion rates measured during life, *J. Clin. Invest.*, 52, 235, 1973.
47. **Casdorph, H. R., Juergens, J. L., Orvis, A. L., and Owen, C. A., Jr.**, Rate of disappearance of cholesterol-^{14}C from the bloodstream of dogs, *Proc. Soc. Exp. Biol. Med.*, 112, 191, 1963.
48. **Chobanian, A. V., Burrows, B. A., and Hollander, W.**, Body cholesterol metabolism in man. II. Measurement of the body cholesterol miscible pool and turnover rate, *J. Clin. Invest.*, 41, 1738, 1962.
49. **Avigan, J., Steinberg, D., and Berman, M.**, Distrbution of labeled cholesterol in animal tissues, *J. Lipid Res.*, 3, 216, 1962.
50. **Nilsson, A. and Zilversmit, D. B.**, Fate of intravenously administered particulate and lipoprotein cholesterol in the rat, *J. Lipid Res.*, 13, 32, 1972.
51. **Farkas, J., Angel, A., and Avigan, M. I.**, Studies on the compartmentation of lipid in adipose cells. II. Cholesterol accumulation and distribution in adipose tissue components, *J. Lipid Res.*, 14, 344, 1973.
52. **Schreibman, P. H. and Dell, R. B.**, Human adipocyte cholesterol: concentration, localization, synthesis, and turnover, *J. Clin. Invest.*, 55, 986, 1975.
53. **Hruza, A. and Zbuzkova, V.**, Cholesterol turnover in plasma, aorta, muscles and erythrocytes in young and old rats, *Mech. Aging and Dev.*, 4, 169, 1975.
54. **Field, H., Jr., Swell, L., Schools, P. E., Jr., and Treadwell, C. R.**, Dynamic aspects of cholesterol metabolism in different areas of the aorta and other tissues in man and their relationship to atherosclerosis, *Circulation*, 22, 547, 1960.
55. **Dayton, S.**, Turnover of cholesterol in the artery walls of normal chickens, *Circ. Res.*, 7, 468, 1959.
56. **Moutafis, C. D. and Myant, N. B.**, The distribution of ^{14}C cholesterol in muscle and skin of rhesus monkeys after intravenous injection, *Clin. Sci. and Mol. Med.*, 50, 307, 1976.
57. **Bhattacharya, A. K., Conner, W. E., Mausolf, F. A., and Flatt, A. E.**, Turnover of Xanthoma cholesterol in hyperlipoproteinemia patients, *J. Lab. Clin. Med.*, 88, 503, 1976.
58. **Smith, F. R., Dell, R. B., Noble, R. P., and Goodman, D. S.**, Parameters of the three-pool model of the turnover of plasma cholesterol in normal and hyperlipidemic humans, *J. Clin. Invest.*, 57, 137, 1976.
59. **Miller, N. E., Nestel, P. J., and Clifton-Bligh, P.**, Relationships between plasma lipoprotein cholesterol concentrations and the pool size and metabolism of cholesterol in man, *Athersclerosis*, 23, 535, 1976.
60. **Bhattacharya, A. K., Conner, W. E., and Spector, A. A.**, Abnormalities of cholesterol turnover in hypercholesterolemic (Type II) patients, *J. Lab. Clin. Med.*, 88, 202, 1976.
61. **Grundy, S. M., Ahrens, E. H., Jr., Salen, G., Schreibman, P. H., and Nestel, P. J.**, Mechanisms of action of clofibrate on cholesterol metabolism in patients with hyperlipidemia, *J. Lipid Res.*, 13, 531, 1972.
62. **Sodhi, H. D., Kudchodkar, J., and Horlick, L.**, Hypocholesterolemic agents and mobilization of tissue cholesterol in man, *Atherosclerosis*, 17, 1, 1973.
63. **Schreibman, P. H. and Ahrens, E. H., Jr.**, Sterol balance in hyperlipidemic patients after dietary exchange of carbohydrate for fat, *J. Lipid Res.*, 17, 97, 1976.
64. **Nestel, P. J., Schreibman, P. H., and Ahrens, E. H., Jr.**, Cholesterol metabolism in human obesity, *J. Clin. Invest.*, 52, 2389, 1973.
65. **Balasubramaniam, S., Mitropoulos, K. A., and Myant, N. B.**, Evidence for the compartmentation of cholesterol in rat liver microsomes, *Eur. J. Biochem.*, 34, 77, 1973.
66. **Ogura, M., Shiga, J., and Yamasaki, K.**, Studies on the cholesterol pool as the precursor of bile acids in the rat, *J. Biochem.*, 70, 967, 1971.
67. **Mitropoulos, K. A., Myant, N. B., Gibbons, G. F., Balasubramaniam, S., and Reeves, E. A.**, Cholesterol precursor pools for the synthesis of cholic and chenodeoxycholic acids in rats, *J. Biol. Chem.*, 249, 6052, 1974.
68. **Schwartz, C. C., Vlahcevic, Z. R., Halloran, L. G., Gregory, D. H., Meek, J. B., and Swell, L.**, Evidence for the existence of definitive hepatic cholesterol precursor compartments for bile acids and biliary cholesterol in man, *Gastroenterology*, 69, 1379, 1975.

69. **Kim, D. N., Lee, K. T., Reiner, J. M., and Thomas, W. A.,** An evaluation of some of the potential immediate sources of cholesterol for bile acid synthesis in swine, *Exp. Mol. Path.*, 22, 284, 1975.
70. **Berman, M.,** Kinetic analysis of turnover data, *Prog. Biochem. Pharmacol.*, 15, 67, 1979.
71. **Schwartz, C. C., Berman, M., Vlahcevic, Z. R., Halloran, L. G., Greogry, D. H., and Swell, L.,** Multicompartmental analysis of cholesterol metabolism in man, *J. Clin. Invest.*, 61, 408, 1978.
72. **Clow, D. J., Dupont, J., Lumb, W. V., Butterfield, A. B., O'Deen, L. A., Oh, S. Y., and Mahoney, T. A.,** Dietary fat and kinetics of cholesterol metabolism in miniature swine. (Unpublished).
73. **Mahoney, T. A.,** Serum lipoprotein cholesterol kinetics, M. S. Thesis, Morgan Library, Colorado State University, Fort Collins, 1975.
74. **Brown, M. S., Goldstein, J. L., Krieger, M., Ho, Y, K., and Anderson, R. G. W.,** Reversible accumulation of cholesteryl esters in macrophages incubated with acetylated lipoproteins, *J. Cell Biol.*, 82, 597, 1979.

INDEX

D

E

F

G

H

I

J

K

L

M

N

O

P

Q

R

S

T

U

V

W

X

Y

Z